Allyn and Bacon

Health on the Net

2002 Edition

Michael Olpin
Weber State University

Doug Gotthoffer
California State University–Northridge

Allyn and Bacon
Boston • London • Toronto • Sydney • Tokyo • Singapore

NOTICE: Between the time Web site information is gathered and then published, it is not unusual for some sites to have ceased operating. Also, the transcription of URLs can result in unintended typographical errors. The Publisher would appreciate notification where these occcur so that they may be corrected in subsequent editions. Thank you.

In its effort to provide a diverse list of Web sites, the Publisher has included links that do not necessarily represent the views of Allyn and Bacon. Faculty, students, and researchers are strongly advised to use their analytical skills to determine the truth, accuracy, and value of the content in individual Web sites.

TRADEMARK CREDITS: Where information was available, trademarks and registered trademarks are indicated below. When detailed information was not available, the publisher has indicated trademark status with an initial capital where those names appear in the text.

Macintosh is a registered trademark of Apple Computer, Inc.

Microsoft is a registered trademark of Microsoft Corporation. Windows, Windows95, Windows98, and Microsoft Internet Explorer are trademarks of Microsoft Corporation.

Netscape and the Netscape Communicator logo are registered trademarks of Netscape Communications Corporation.

A Pearson Education Company
75 Arlington Street
Boston, MA 02116
Internet: www.ablongman.com

ISBN 0-205-34669-3

Printed in the United States of America

10 9 8 7 6 5 4 3 2 1 03 02 01

Contents

Part 1 Introduction to the Internet

Part 2 Internet Activities for Health

part 1

Introduction to the Internet

You're about to embark on an exciting experience as you become one of the millions of citizens of the Internet. Once you've accustomed yourself to this wonderful new world, you'll be amazed by how much you can discover, learn, and accomplish as you explore the Internet's dynamic resources.

Why Use the Internet?

In *Understanding Media,* Marshall McLuhan foresaw the existence of the Internet when he described electronic media as an extension of our central nervous system. On the other hand, today's students introduced to the Internet for the first time describe it as "cool."

No matter which description you favor, you are immersed in a period that is transforming the way we live by transforming the nature of the information we live by. As recently as 1980, intelligence was marked by "knowing things." If you were born in that year, by the time you were old enough to cross the street by yourself, that definition had changed radically. Today, in a revolution that makes McLuhan's vision tangible, events, facts, rumors, and gossip are distributed instantly to all parts of the global body. The effects are equivalent to a shot of electronic adrenaline. No longer the domain of the privileged few, information is shared by all the inhabitants of McLuhan's global village. Meanwhile, the concept of information as intelligence feels as archaic as a television remote control with a wire on it (ask your parents about that).

With hardly more effort than it takes to rub your eyes open in the morning, you can connect with the latest news, gossip about your favorite music group or TV star, learn the best places to eat on spring break, find out the weather back home, or follow the trials and tribulations of that soap opera character whose life conflicts with your history class. You can carry on a real-time conversation with your best friend at a college half a continent away, or play interactive games with a dozen or more world-wide challengers. And that's just for fun. When it comes to your education, newspaper and magazine archives are now almost instantly available, as are the contents of many reference books. Distant and seemingly unapproachable experts are found answering questions in discussion groups or electronic newsletters.

The Internet also addresses the major problem facing us in our split-second, efficiency-rated culture: Where do we find the time? The Internet allows professors and students to keep in touch, collaborate, and learn without placing unreasonable demands on individual schedules. Professors are posting everything from course syllabi to homework solutions and are increasingly answering questions online, all in an effort to ease the pressure for face-to-face meetings by supplementing them with cyberspace offices. The Internet enables students and professors to expand office hours into a twenty-four-hours-a-day, seven-days-a-week operation. Many classes have individual sites at which enrolled students can gather electronically to swap theories, ideas, resources, gripes, and triumphs.

By freeing us from the more mundane operations of information gathering, and by providing numerous diverse sources of information, the Internet encourages us to be more creative and imaginative. Instead of devoting most of our time to gathering information and precious little to analyzing and synthesizing it, the Internet tips the balance in favor of the skills that separate us from silicon chips. As much as the Internet ties us together, it simultaneously emphasizes our individual skills—our ability to connect information in new, meaningful, and exciting ways. Rarely have we had the opportunity to make connections and observations on such a wide range of topics, to create more individual belief systems, and to chart a path through learning that makes information personally useful and meaningful.

A Brief History of the Internet

The Internet began as a tool for national defense. In the mid-1960s, the U.S. Department of Defense was searching for an information analogy to the new Interstate Highway System, a way to move computing resources around the country in the event the Cold War caught fire. The immediate predicament, however, had to do with the Defense Department's budget, and the millions of dollars spent on computer research at universities and think tanks. Much of these millions was spent on acquiring, building, or modifying large computer systems to meet the demands of the emerging fields of computer graphics, artificial intelligence, and multiprocessing (where one computer was shared among dozens of different tasks).

While the research was distributed across the country, the unwieldy, often temperamental, computers were not. This made it difficult for computer scientists at various institutions to share their work without duplicating each other's hardware. Wary of being accused of re-inventing the wheel, the Advanced Research Projects Agency (ARPA), the funding arm of the Defense Department, invested in the ARPANET, a private network that would allow disparate computer systems to communicate with each other. Researchers could remain among their colleagues at their home campuses while using computing resources at government research sites thousands of miles away.

A small group of ARPANET citizens soon began writing computer programs to perform little tasks across the Internet. Most of these programs, while ostensibly meeting immediate research needs, were written for the challenge of writing them. These programmers, for example, created the first email systems. They also created games such as "Space Wars" and "Adventure." Driven in large part by the novelty and practicality of email, businesses and institutions accepting government research funds begged and borrowed their way onto the ARPANET, and the number of connections swelled.

As the innocence of the 1960s gave way to the business sense of the 1980s, the government eased out of the networking business, turning the ARPANET (now Internet) over to its users. While we capitalize the word "Internet," it may surprise you to learn there is no "Internet, Inc." in charge of this uniquely postmodern creation. Administration of this world-wide communication complex is still handled by the cooperating institutions and regional networks that comprise the Internet. The word "Internet" denotes a specific interconnected network of networks, not a corporate entity.

The emergence of the World Wide Web, developed by the European Laboratory for Particle Physics in the early 1990s, transformed the Internet. For the first time, images as well as text could be viewed through the aid of graphical Web browsers (software for navigating the Web).

Today, sophisticated browsers such as Netscape Navigator and Microsoft Internet Explorer have led to the Web's vast popularity.

Some Things You Ought to Know

In order to access the Internet, you must first have an Internet Service Provider (ISP). That's the organization providing you with your Internet account. Most of the time your ISP will be your school; but you may contract with one of the commercial providers such as America Online, the Microsoft Network, Earthlink, or AT&T.

Much of the confusion over the Internet comes from two sources. One is terminology. Just as the career you're preparing for has its own special vocabulary, so does the Internet. You'd be hard pressed to join in the shoptalk of archeologists, librarians, or carpenters if you didn't speak their language. Don't expect to plop yourself down in the middle of the Internet without some buzzwords under your belt, either. This chapter will explain the most common terms, but keep in mind that new Internet technologies are developing all the time.

The second source of confusion is that there are often many ways to accomplish the same ends on the Internet. This is a direct by-product of the freedom so highly cherished by Net citizens. When someone has an idea for doing something, he or she puts it out there and lets the Internet community decide its merits. As a result, it's difficult to put down in writing the *one exact* way to send email, search for information, or whatever.

There are also differences in the workings of a PC or Mac and the various versions of the two major Web browsers, Netscape and Microsoft Internet Explorer. If you can't find a particular command or function mentioned in the book, chances are it's there, but in a different place or with a slightly different name. Check the manual or online help that came with your computer, or ask a more computer-savvy friend or professor.

If learning about the Internet is making you a little nervous, relax! Getting up to speed takes a little time, but the effort will be well rewarded. Approach learning your way around the Internet with the same enthusiasm and curiosity you approach learning your way around a new college campus. This isn't a competition. Nobody's keeping score. And the only winner will be you.

Introducing the World Wide Web

If you've never seriously used the Web, you are about to take your first steps on what can only be described as an incredible journey. Just as no one owns the Internet, there is no formal organization among the collection of hundreds of thousands of computers that make up the part of the Net called the World Wide Web.

Initially, you might find it convenient to think of the Web as cable television with millions of channels. It's safe to say that, among all these channels, there's something for you to watch. Only, how do you find it? You could click through the channels one by one, of course, but by the time you found something of interest it would either (1) be over or (2) leave you wondering if there wasn't something better on that you're missing.

A more efficient way to search for what you want would be to consult some sort of TV listing. While you could skim through pages more rapidly than channels, the task would still be daunting. A more creative approach would allow you to press a button on your remote control that would connect you to a channel of interest; what's more, that channel would contain the names (or numbers) of other channels with similar programs. Those channels in turn would contain information about other channels. Now you could zip through this million-channel universe, touching down only at programs of potential interest.

If you have a feel for how this might work for television, you have a feel for what it's like to journey around (or "surf") the Web. Instead of channels, we have *Web sites*. Each site contains one or more *pages*. Each page may contain links to other pages, either in the same site or in other sites, anywhere in the world. These other pages may elaborate on the information you're looking at, direct you to related but not identical information, or even provide contrasting or contradictory points of view. And, of course, these pages could have links of their own.

Today, Web sites are maintained by businesses, institutions, affinity groups, professional organizations, government departments, and ordinary people anxious to express opinions, share information, sell products, or provide services. Because these sites are stored electronically, updating them is more convenient and practical than updating printed media. That makes Web sites far more dynamic than other types of research material you may be used to, and it means a visit to a Web site can open up new opportunities that weren't available as recently as a few hours ago.

Hypertext and Links

The invention that unveils these revolutionary possibilities is called *hypertext.* Hypertext is a technology for combining text, graphics, sounds, video, and links on a single World Wide Web page. Unlike traditional linear documents such as books, hypertext allows navigation through pages in any order that you like. Click on a link and you're transported, like Alice falling down the rabbit hole, to a new page, a new address, a new environment for research and communication.

Links come in three flavors: text, picture, and hot spot. A text link may be a letter, a word, a phrase, a sentence, or any contiguous combination of text characters. You can identify text links at a glance because the characters are underlined and often displayed in a unique color, setting the link apart from the rest of the text on the page. Picture links may be drawings, photos, or other graphic elements. On the Web, a picture may not only be worth a thousand words, but also the start of a journey into a whole new corner of cyberspace.

The hot spot is neither underlined nor bordered. It would be impossible to see were it not for a Web convention that offers you (literally) a helping hand for finding all types of links. Whenever the mouse cursor

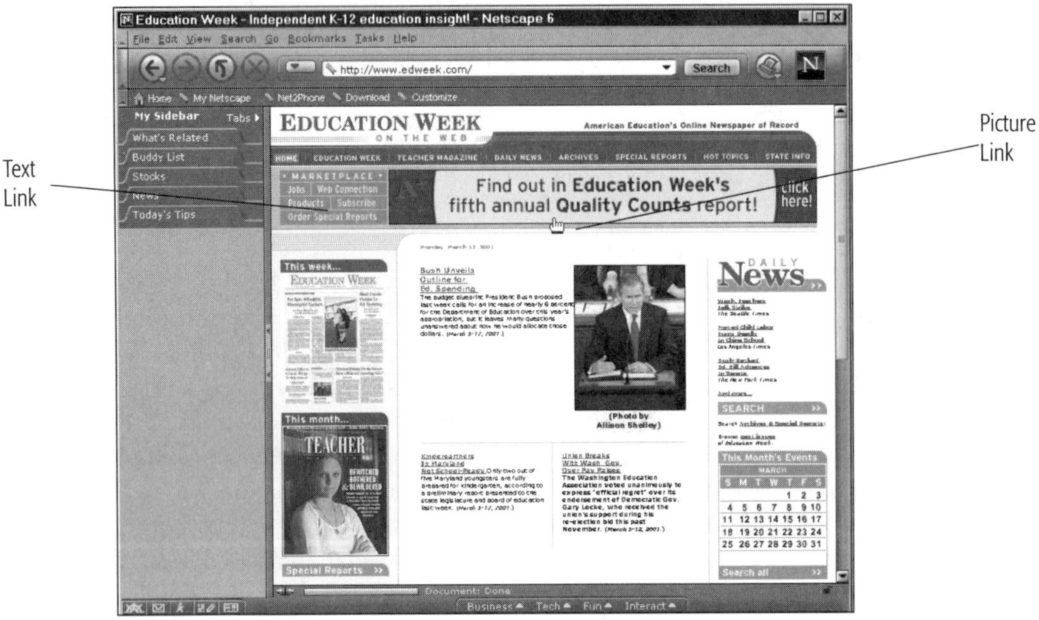

Text links are underlined and set off in color. You can tell this picture is a link because the mouse cursor has changed from an arrow to a hand.

passes over a link, the cursor changes from an arrow to a hand. Wherever you see the hand icon, you can click and retrieve another Web page. Sweep the cursor over an area of interest, see the hand, follow the link, and you're surfing the Web. Hot spots are sometimes located on areas of a large picture called an "image map." Clicking on different areas of the image map will lead you to different Web pages.

In the Name of the Page

Zipping around the Web in this way may seem exciting, even serendipitous, but it's also fraught with peril. How, for instance, do you revisit a page of particular interest? Or share a page with a classmate? Or cite a page as a reference for a professor? Web page designers assign titles to their pages; unfortunately, there's nothing to prevent two designers from assigning the same title to different pages.

An instrument that uniquely identifies Web pages does exist. It's called a *Universal Resource Locator (URL).* A URL contains all the information necessary to locate the:

- Web page containing the information you're looking for;
- computer that hosts (stores) that page of information;
- form in which the information is stored.

A typical URL looks like this:

```
http://www.abacon.com/index.html
```

You enter it into the **Location** or **Address** field at the top of your browser window. Hit the **Return** (or **Enter**) key, and your browser will deliver to your screen the exact page specified. When you click on a link, you're actually using a shorthand alternative to typing the URL yourself because the browser does it for you. In fact, if you watch the "Location" or "Address" field when you click on a link, you'll see its contents change to the URL to which you're traveling.

The URL Exposed

How does your browser know where you're going? As arcane as the URL appears, there is a logical explanation to its apparent madness. This is true not only of URLs, but also of computers in general. Because a computer's "intelligence" only extends to following simple instructions exactly, most of the commands, instructions, and procedures you'll encounter have simple underlying patterns. Once you familiarize yourself with these patterns, you'll find you're able to make major leaps in your understanding of new Internet features.

To unscramble the mysteries of Web addresses, we'll start at the end of the URL and work our way toward the front.

```
/index.html
```

This is the name of a single file or document. Eventually, the contents of this file/document will be transferred over the Internet to your computer. However, because there are undoubtedly thousands of files on the Internet with this name, we need to clarify our intentions a bit more.

```
www.abacon.com
```

This is the name of a particular Internet *Web server,* a computer whose job it is to forward Web pages to you on request. By Internet convention, this name is unique. The combination of

```
www.abacon.com/index.html
```


identifies a unique file/document on a unique Web server on the World Wide Web. No other file has this combined address, so there's no question about which file/document to transfer to you.

The characters *http://* at the beginning of the URL identify the method by which the file/document will be transferred. The letters stand for HyperText Transfer Protocol.

You Can Go Home (and to Other Pages) Again

You know that a URL uniquely identifies a Web page and that links let you travel from page to page, but what if you end up at a dead end? Missing page messages take several forms, such as "URL 404," "Object not on this server," "Missing Object," or "Page Not Found," but they all tell you that the page specified by the link or URL no longer exists.

There are many reasons for missing pages. You may have entered the URL incorrectly (every character must be precise and no spaces are allowed). More than likely, though, especially if you arrived here via a link, the page you're after has been moved or removed. Remember, anybody can create a link to any page. That's the good news. The bad news is that the owner of a page is under no obligation to inform the owners of links pointing to it that the page location has changed. In fact, there's no way for the page owner to even know about all the links to that page. Yes, the Internet's spirit of independence proves frustrating sometimes, but you'll

Quick Check

Don't Be Lost In (Hyper)Space

Let's pause for a quick check of your Web navigation skills. Look at the sample Web page below. How many links does it contain?

Did you find four? The four links include:

1. The word "links" in the second line below the seaside picture;
2. The sentence "What about me?";
3. The word "cyberspace" in the quick brown fox sentence;
4. The hot spot in the seaside picture. We know there's at least one link in the picture, because the cursor appears as a hand. (There may be more hot spots on the page, but we can't tell from this picture alone.)

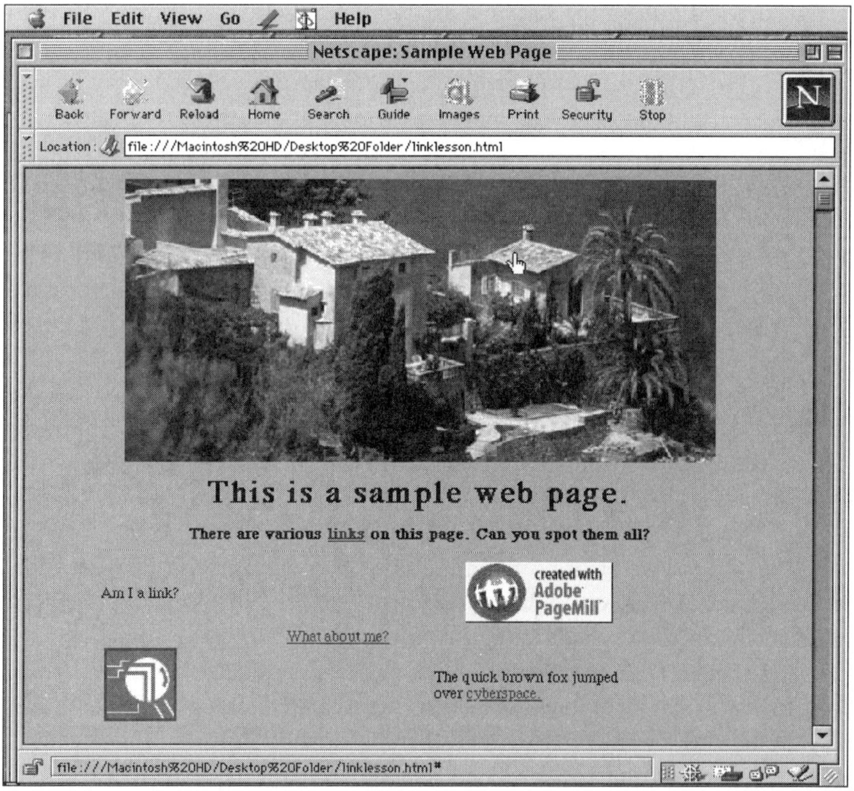

A sample web page to exercise your link identifying skills.

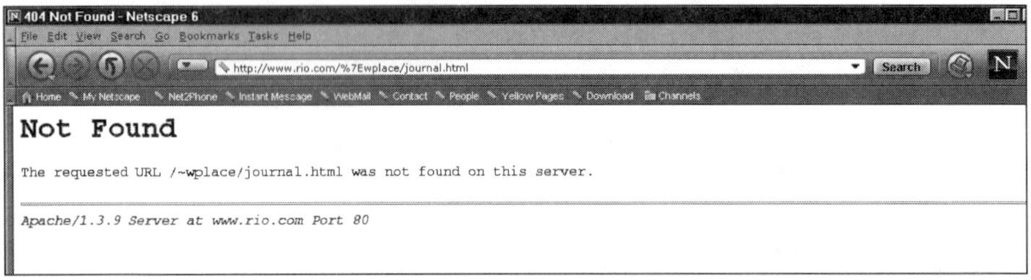

A missing page message, an all too common road hazard on the information superhighway.

find these small inconveniences are a cheap price to pay for the benefits you receive. Philosophy aside, though, we're still stuck on a page of no interest to us. The best strategy is to back up and try another approach.

Every time you click on the **Back** button (or back arrow in Netscape 6) at the top of the browser, you return to the previous page visited. That's because your browser keeps track of the pages you visit and the order in which you visit them. The **Back** button, and its counterpart, the **Forward** button (or forward arrow in Netscape 6), allow you to retrace the steps of your cyberpath.

What if you want to move two, three, or a dozen pages at once? Although you can click the **Back** or **Forward** buttons multiple times, Web browsers offer an easier navigation shortcut. If you use Netscape, clicking on the **Go** menu in the menu bar displays a list of your most recently visited pages, in the order in which you visited them. Unlike the **Back** or **Forward** buttons, you can select any page from the menu, and a single click takes you directly there. There's no need to laboriously move one page a time. If you use Internet Explorer, you can click on the **History** button in the Explorer bar or press the arrow at the end of the Address bar to see a list of links you visited in previous days and weeks.

Suppose you want to return to a page hours, days, or even months later. One way is to write down the URL of every page you may want to revisit. There's got to be a better way, and there is: We call them *bookmarks* (in Netscape) or *favorites* (in Microsoft Internet Explorer).

Like their print book namesakes, bookmarks (and favorites) flag specific Web pages. Selecting an item from the **Bookmark/Favorites** menu, like selecting an item from the **Go** menu, is the equivalent of entering a URL into the **Location** field of your browser, except that items in the **Bookmark/Favorites** menu are ones you've added yourself and represent pages visited over many surfing experiences, not just the most recent one.

In Netscape 6, to save a favorite Web page, pull down the **Bookmarks** menu and click on the **Add Current Page** command. When you want to select a page from your bookmark list, just click on the desired entry. To edit the title or URL of a bookmark, choose **Manage Bookmarks.** This feature also lets you arrange your favorites in folders by category.

Selecting **Add to Favorites** from the **Favorites** menu performs the same function as Bookmarks in Netscape 6 and adds the location of the current page to your list of favorite pages. If you want to be able to review this page when you're not online, click on the "Make available offline" checkbox.

A cautionary note is in order here. Your Bookmark or Favorites list physically exists only on your personal computer, which means that if you connect to the Internet on a different computer, your list won't be available. However, if you routinely connect to the Internet from a computer lab, there is a way to avoid the work of retyping your URLs each time you use a different computer. Both Internet Explorer and Netscape provide procedures to save favorites in a computer file that you can move from one computer to another. You can export a selected folder in your Favorites list, or all of your favorites. Since exported favorites are saved as an HTML file, either Internet Explorer or Navigator can import them.

In Internet Explorer 5.5, under the File menu, choose **Import and Export** to pull up the Import/Export Wizard. Follow the on-screen instructions to **Export Favorites.** You will see a list of files. Insert a blank diskette into the diskette drive and choose the diskette drive on which you want to export the favorites. When you begin working on a different computer, insert your diskette with the file of favorites into the diskette drive. Again choose Import and Export from the File menu and follow the on-screen instructions to **Import Favorites.** Click on Browse to indicate where you want to import the favorites.

In Netscape 6, click on **Bookmarks,** and then **Manage Bookmarks.** Then, in the window that opens, select **Export Bookmarks** from under the File menu. A list of files on your hard drive will appear. Insert a blank diskette and click on the arrow beside the "Save in" prompt to change the drive. When you begin working on a different computer, insert your diskette with the file of bookmarks into the diskette drive. Again, click on Bookmarks, Manage Bookmarks, and select **Import Bookmarks** from the File menu. Locate the filename of your bookmarks in the browser window and open it. Your bookmark file will now open when you choose Bookmarks.

Quick Check

As a quick review, here's what we know about navigating the Web so far:

- Enter a URL directly into the Location field;
- Click on a link;
- Use the **Back** or **Forward** icons;
- Select a page from the **Go** menu.
- Add bookmarks or favorite URLs.

Searching and Search Engines

Returning to our cable television analogy, you may recall that we glossed over the question of how we selected a starting channel in the first place. With a million TV channels, or several million Web pages, we can't depend solely on luck guiding us to something interesting.

On the Web, we solve the problem with specialized computer programs called *search engines* that crawl through the Web, page by page, cataloging its contents. As different software designers developed search strategies, entrepreneurs established Web sites where any user could find pages containing particular words and phrases. Today, Web sites such as Yahoo! offer you a "front door" to the Internet that begins with a search for content of interest.

The URLs for some popular search sites are:

AltaVista	`www.altavista.com`
Excite	`www.excite.com`
Google	`www.google.com`
HotBot	`www.hotbot.lycos.com`
Infoseek	`www.infoseek.com`
MetaCrawler	`www.metacrawler.com`

WebCrawler	`www.webcrawler.com`
Yahoo!	`www.yahoo.com`

Internet Gold Is Where You Find It

Let's perform a simple search using Hotbot to find information about the history of the Internet. See the results in the screen shown below and on pages 14–16.

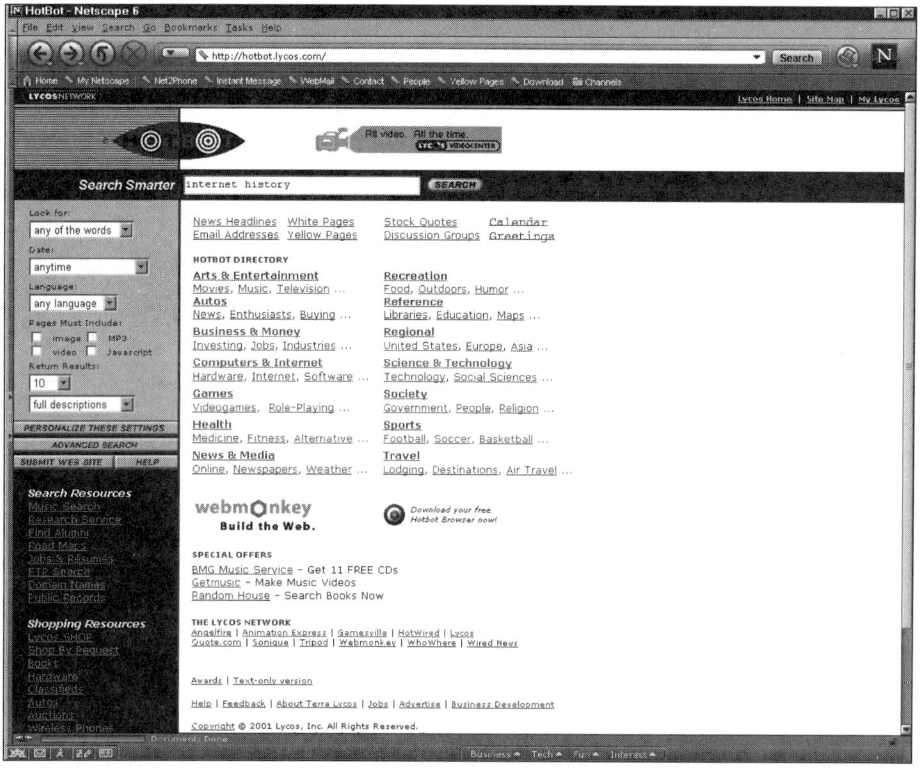

We'll start by searching for the words "internet" or "history." By looking for "any of the words," the search will return pages on which either "internet" or "history" or both appear.

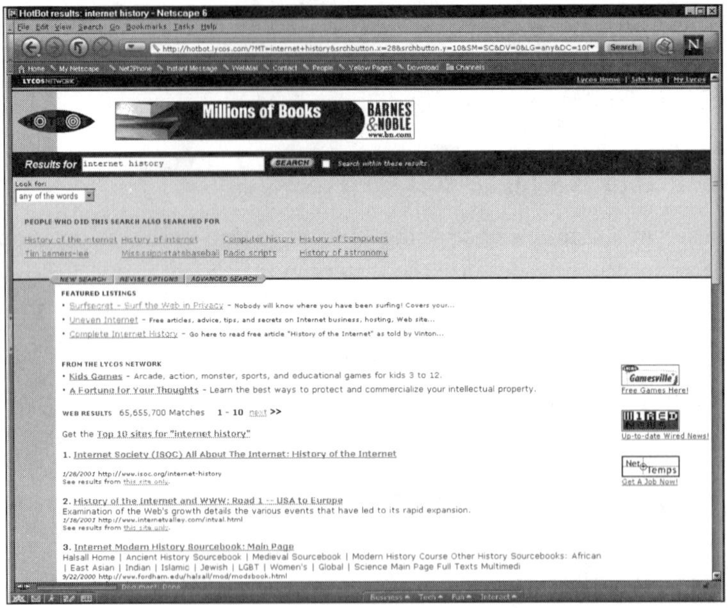

part
1

Our search returned more than 50 million matches or *hits*. Pages are ranked according to the following factors: words in the title, keyword meta tags, word frequency in the document, and document length.

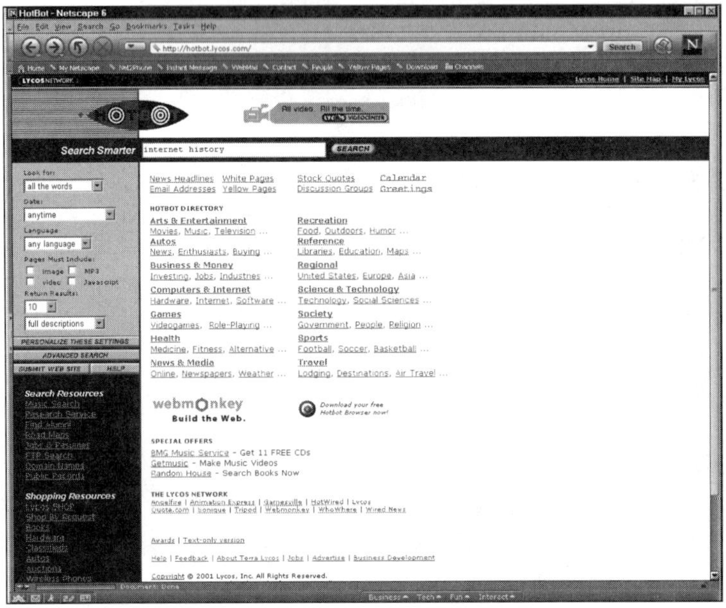

We can conduct the same search, but this time look for "all the words." The search will return hits when both "internet" and "history" appear on the same page, in any order, and not necessarily next to each other.

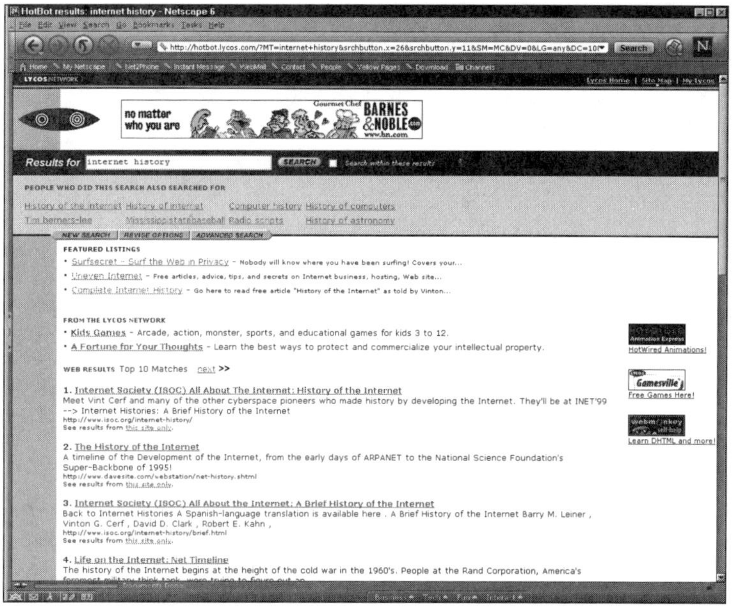

The search is narrowed down somewhat, but still has more than 5 million hits. You'll note that HotBot has provided a Top 10 list of results for this search.

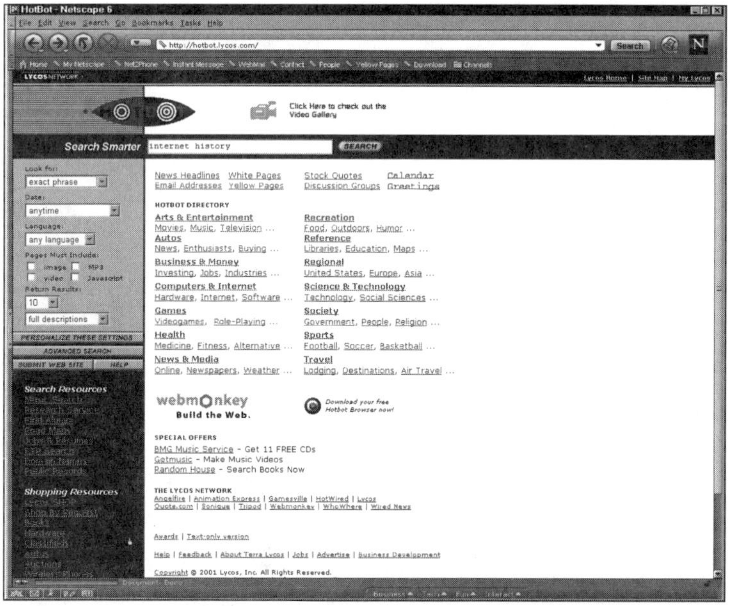

When we search for the exact phrase "internet history," which means those two words in exactly that order, with no intervening words, we're down to several thousand hits (still a substantial number).

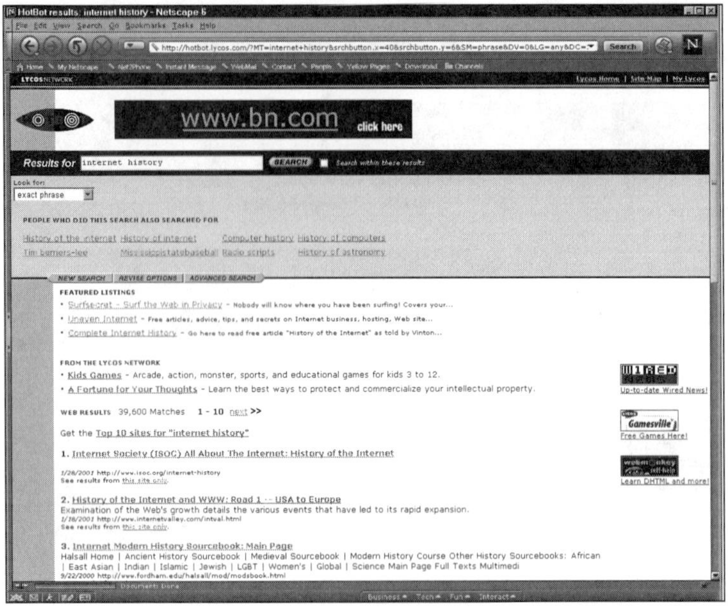

Now the first hits may be more specific. However, other hits in the list may have nothing to do with the history of the Internet. Hits happen. No search engine is 100 percent accurate 100 percent of the time. Spurious search results are the serendipity of the Internet. Look at them as an opportunity to explore something new.

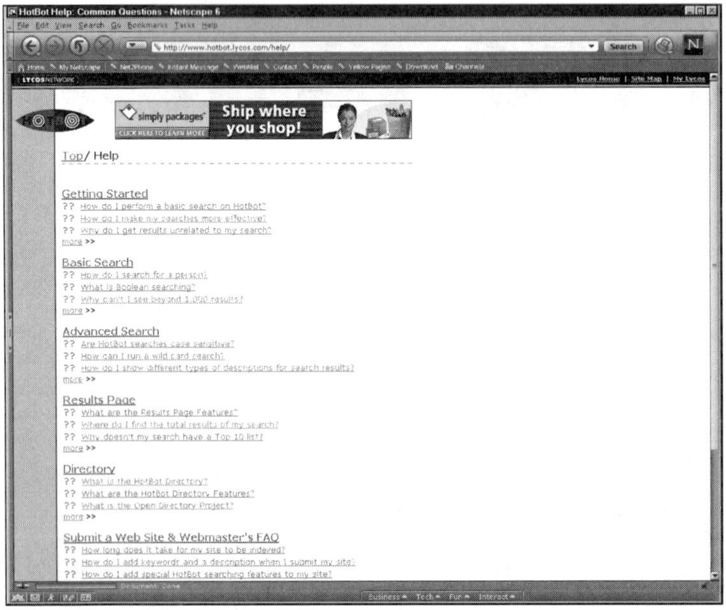

Clearly, narrowing down your search as much as possible is essential. Click on Help in the Search area on the left side of the HotBot page to obtain tips for narrowing your search. You'll find search tip pages like this at all the major search engine sites.

Out of curiosity, let's try our history of the Internet search using a different search engine. When we search for the phrase "history of the internet" using WebCrawler, the quotation marks serve the same purpose as selecting "the exact phrase" option in HotBot. But the WebCrawler search only finds approximately 900 hits. Some are the same as those found using HotBot, some are different. Different searching strategies and software algorithms make using more than one search engine a must for serious researchers.

The major search engines conveniently provide you with tips to help you get the most out of their searches. These include ways to use AND and OR to narrow down searches, and ways to use NOT to eliminate unwanted hits.

Each search engine also uses a slightly different approach to cataloging the Web, so your results may vary. Often, one search engine provides better results (more relevant hits) in your areas of interest; sometimes the wise strategy is to provide the same input to several different engines. No one search engine does a perfect job all the time, so experience will dictate the one that's most valuable to you.

Quick Check

Let's review our searching strategies:

- Visit one of the search engine sites;
- Enter key words or phrases that best describe the search criteria;
- Narrow the search if necessary by using options such as "all the words" or "the exact phrase." On some search engines, you may use the word "and" or the symbol "|" to indicate words that all must appear on a page;
- Try using the same criteria with different search engines.

Additional Internet Resources

Developed by the University of Minnesota, **Gopher** was an early method for navigating the Internet. Where did it get its name? Some say a gopher was the university's mascot, but the name also sounds like "go for." And what you go for are files at a Gopher site. The contents are listed in a hierarchical menu with folders containing files. Text files can be read in a window. Gopher sites are still run by some universities. You can use your Web browser to connect by typing gopher://*name of site* in the location box.

Telnet is a program used to access remote databases, library catalogs, and MUDs/MOOs (discussed later in this chapter). Telnet uses Unix commands and is not very user-friendly. Some universities have telnet sites that require you to have an account on their server. Other sites let you log in as a guest. You can access a telnet site with your Web browser by typing telnet://*address of site*. A menu of options will appear.

File Transfer Protocol (FTP) is a method for sending (*uploading*) and receiving (*downloading*) files over the Internet. These files may be free software, text, graphics, audio, or video. Anonymous FTP sites allow anyone to log in as "anonymous" and use an email address as a password. For a list of FTP sites and tutorials, see FTPplanet.com at www.ftpplanet.com.

To access an FTP site with your Web browser, just enter the address in the location box by typing ftp://*address of site*. Once you are connected, you will see a directory listing with folder icons and document files. Special FTP client programs make it easy to send and receive files, or to transfer more than one file at a time. They are often used for managing Web sites. An example is WS_FTP, which you can download at www.ipswitch.com/pd_wsftp.html.

Plug-Ins Bring the Web to Life

Plug-ins are free software that allow Web pages to include audio, video, or animation. Some plug-ins, such as RealPlayer (audio and video) and Netscape Radio (live radio), are now included with Netscape. Others must be downloaded and installed before they can be used. These files may be compressed and need a utility program such as WinZip for Windows (www.winzip.com) or Stuffit for the Mac (www.aladdinsys.com) to decompress them.

Here are five plug-ins and where to get more information:

- Macromedia ShockWave makes it possible to view complex animations and engage in interactions with the software. See www.macromedia.com/shockwave.
- RealAudio compresses audio files and transmits them over the Internet. It uses a technique called "streaming audio" so that the

sound will start to play while the file is still downloading. The RealAudio Player appears in a separate window on your monitor. See www.realaudio.com.

- QuickTime Video was developed by Apple Computer, Inc. The QuickTime Player lets you play video files. There are versions for both the PC and the Mac. See quicktime.apple.com.
- The Macromedia Flash Viewer enables you to view animated text or graphics. It is also used for animated slide shows, games, and educational interactions. See www.macromedia.com.
- The Adobe Acrobat Viewer lets you view and print files created in Adobe Portable Document Format, a way of storing pages with complex layout. See www.adobe.com/products/acrobat/readermain.html.

Give Your Web Browser Some Personality—Yours

Email and newsgroups let you communicate with others through the Internet at your own pace and on your own time. Before you can access these functions, however, you must set up or personalize your browser. If you always work on the same computer, this is a one-time operation in which you tell your browser where to find essential computer servers, along with personal information the Internet needs to move messages for you.

Begin by setting up your desired home page. This is the page that you will see whenever you first log on to the Internet. You can return to this page at any time by clicking on the **Home** icon. For example, for your convenience, you may want your browser to start by fetching your favorite search site or your school library's home page. Both Netscape 6 and Internet Explorer 5.5 offer the option of a blank home page. In that case, you will get a blank browser window.

To set up your home page in Netscape 6, go to the **Edit** menu and click on **Preferences.** Type in the URL of the page you want to use as your home page. The Appearance tab lets you set up Web preferences such as the color of links and visited links (the default is blue and purple), style and size of fonts, themes (look of buttons and toolbars) history (how long to keep a list of pages you've visited), the layout of mail and newsgroups messages, and advanced options. In Internet Explorer 5.5, you can set up a home page through the **Internet Options** found under the **Tools** menu.

Next, set up your browser for mail and newsgroup operation. You need to know the name of the mail and news servers along with your user name and other details, such as the address of the domain name server (DNS) of your ISP. You should have received all this information when you opened your Internet account. If not, ask for it. Help provided by the Windows and Mac operating systems will automatically enter some of this information for you.

Netscape 6 differs from earlier versions of this browser in that it makes it possible to set up several email accounts using different servers. Each account has a separate inbox for receiving mail. For each account, you create an account name and server settings such as server type, server name, user name, and port. An area for mail folders appears on the left, while an area for a list of the mail you've received will appear on the right, including the Subject, Sender, and Date.

To set up your email and newsgroup accounts with Netscape 6, under the **Tasks** menu, select **Mail.** Choose **Edit** and then **Mail/News Account Settings** to activate the Account Wizard. The Account Settings menu will appear. Enter the type of account you want to set up: email, WebMail (Netscape's own email service), America Online, or newsgroup. Enter your name and email address and click on Next. The information you are asked to enter next depends on the type of account you are setting up.

For example, if setting up an email account, be sure to use your user name (and not your alias) in the "Account Name" field. Your Reply To address is typically the same as your email address, though if you have an email alias you can use it here. You can attach a signature such as a favorite saying to each piece of mail you send. You can also choose to write your messages in plain text or in HTML.

Now highlight the **Server** category to tell the browser where to find your mail servers. The SMTP server handles your outgoing messages, while the POP3 or IMAP mail server routes incoming mail. The outgoing SMTP server is usually the same for all accounts, including newsgroups. Indicate how often you want Netscape to check for new messages (the default is every 10 minutes).

To add a new account, click the **New Account** button. Again, select the type of account. For example, if you choose newsgroup, you must enter the name of your news (NNTP) server such as "news.netscape.net" by highlighting the Server category. The Internet Connection Wizard may automatically enter the newsgroup server name your ISP has provided. Again, be sure to specify how often Netscape should check for new messages. If you do not do this, you will have to click on the Get Msg button to retrieve messages.

Click on OK in the bottom right part of the window when finished adding your accounts. This will save the information.

Netscape 6 also lets you choose the font style and color for email and newsgroup messages. Just go to **Edit, Preferences, Mail and Newsgroups,** and then click on **Message Display.** You can choose whether to wrap text or display emoticons (e.g., little smiley faces) as graphics. If you click on **Message Composition,** you can indicate whether you want a message to which you are replying to be quoted within your email and where it will appear. To set up automatic address collection, select **Address Books.**

In Internet Explorer 5.5, the Internet Connection Wizard will help you set up the email server and newsgroup (NNTP) server provided by your ISP. Go to the Tools menu and choose Internet Options. Then click on the Setup button to bring up the wizard. You can view or modify how your server connections are set up by clicking on **Internet Options** under the **Tools** menu. Click on the **Connections** tab and then **Settings and Properties.** Finally, click on **Server Types** for information about your dial-up server to the Internet.

To select an email program to use, from the **Internet Options** window click on **Programs.**A list of email services will come up to choose from, such as Hotmail, Microsoft Outlook, Outlook Express, or America Online. You can also indicate whether you want to use HTML to write your email messages. Then click on **Newsgroups** to select a newsgroup program.

The (E)mail Goes Through

Email was one of the first applications created for the Internet by its designers. Your electronic Internet mailbox is to email what a post office box is to "snail mail" (the name Net citizens apply to ordinary, hand-delivered mail). This mailbox resides on the computer of your ISP. The Internet doesn't deliver a message to your door but instead leaves it in a conveniently accessible place (your mailbox) in the post office (the computer of your ISP), until you retrieve the mail using your combination (password).

If you currently have access to the Internet, your school or ISP assigned you a *username* (also called a user id, account name, or account number). This username may be your first name, your first initial and the first few characters of your last name, or some strange combination of numbers and letters only a computer could love. An email address is a combination of your username and the unique address of the computer through which you access your email. For example:

```
username@computername.edu
```

The three letters after the dot, in this case "edu," identify the top level "domain." There are six common domain categories in use: edu (educational), com (commercial), org (organization), net (network), mil (military), and gov (government). The symbol "@"—called the "at" sign—serves two purposes: For computers, it provides a neat, clean separation between your username and the computer name; for people, it makes Internet addresses more pronounceable. Your address is read: username "at" computer name "dot" e-d-u. Suppose your Internet username is "a4736g" and your ISP is Allyn & Bacon, the publisher of this book. Your email address might look like

```
a4736g@abacon.com
```

and you would tell people your email address is "ay-four-seven-three-six-gee at ay bacon dot com."

We Don't Just Handle Your Email, We're Also a Client

You use email with the aid of special programs called *mail clients*. As with search engines, mail clients have the same set of core features, but your access to these features varies with the type of program. On both the PC and the Mac, Netscape and Microsoft Internet Explorer give you access to mail clients while you're plugged into the Web. That way you can pick up and send mail while you're surfing the Web. The basic email service functions are creating and sending mail, reading mail, replying to mail, and forwarding mail. First we'll examine the process of sending and reading mail, and then we'll discuss how to set up your programs so that your messages arrive safely.

Let's look at a typical mail client screen, in this case from Netscape 6. You reach this screen by choosing **Mail** from the **Tasks** menu. The **Mail Toolbar** appears across the top of the Netscape Mail window. Under the toolbar and to the left appear the folders contained in each email account, such as Inbox, Unsent Messages, Drafts, Sent, and Trash. The Message List window lists the current mail, including the Subject, Sender, and Date. The first message appears in a message window. Click on the Next button to read the next new message. You can choose how to sort messages by choosing **Sort** from the **View** menu.

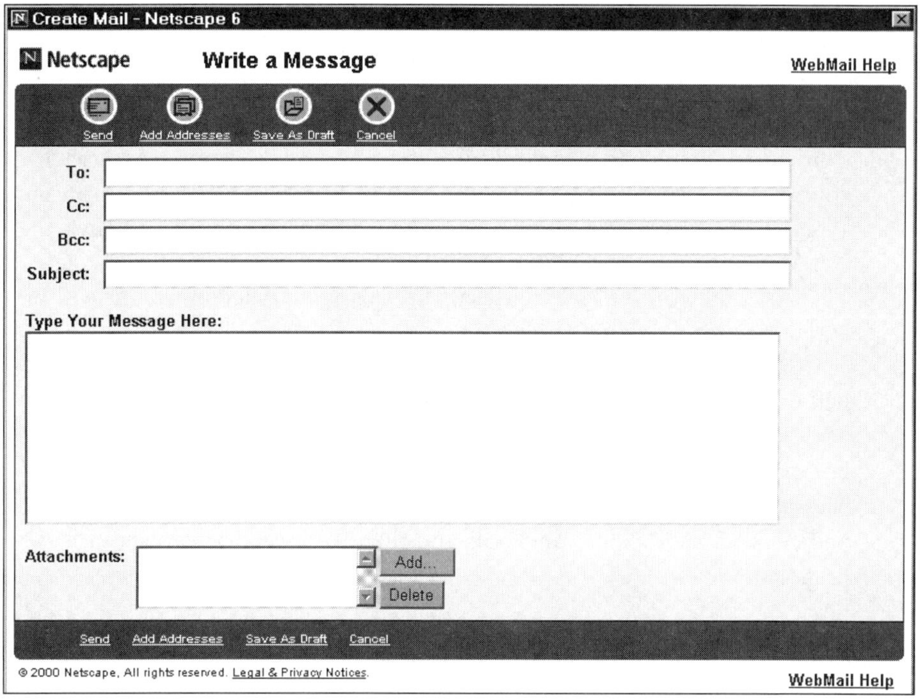

New message form, with fields for recipient's address and the subject, and a window for the text of the message.

To send an email message, from the **File** menu choose **New,** then **Message.** If the mail window is already open, an easier method is to click on the **New Msg** button from the Mail toolbar. This creates a blank Message Compose window that has a "from" field for your address, a "to" field for the recipient's address, a subject field, and a window in which to type the text of the message. Type the address or select a recipient from the automated Address Book by clicking on the **Address** button. You can attach a file to your message with the **Attach** button. To save a copy of your message, click on **Save.**

Fill in the recipient's address in the "To" field, just above the arrow. Use your own address. We'll send email to ourselves and use the same message to practice sending email and reading it as well; then you'll know if your messages come out as expected. Click in the "Subject" field and enter a word or phrase that generally describes the topic of the message. Since we're doing this for the first time, let's type "Maiden Email Voyage." Click anywhere in the text window and enter your message: "Hi. Thanks for guiding me through sending my first email." You'll find that the mail client works here like a word processing program, which means you can insert and delete words and characters and highlight text.

When you've finished the message, click on the **Send** button. You've just created and sent your first email message. In most systems, it takes from a few seconds to a few minutes for a message to yourself to reach your mailbox, so you might want to take a short break before continuing. When you're ready to proceed, close the Compose window and click the **Get Msg** button on the Mail window toolbar to receive your message. The first time you retrieve a message from an email account, you will be asked to enter a password.

In Internet Explorer 5.5, the appearance of the mail client screen will depend on your email program. Pull up the **Tools** menu and select **Mail and News.** This menu lets you read mail or send a new message. For example, to use the Microsoft Express email program, select **New Message** and click on OK to open a message window. Type your message and click on **Send.** Click on **Tools** and then **Address Book** to set up a list of contacts.

What Goes Around Comes Around

Now let's retrieve the message you just sent to yourself. When retrieving mail, most mail clients display a window showing the messages in your mailbox and telling you how many new messages have been added.

If you've never used your email before, chances are that your message window is empty, or contains only one or two messages (usually official messages from the ISP) besides the one you sent to yourself. The message to yourself should be accompanied by an indicator of some sort—such as a closed envelope icon—indicating it's a new message. You also get to see the date of the message, who sent it, and the information you entered in the subject line. The Subject field lets you scan your messages and determine which ones you want to look at first.

The summary of received messages tells you everything you need to know about a message except what's in it. Click anywhere on the line to see the contents in the message window. Click on the message from yourself and you'll see the contents of the message displayed in a window. The information at the top—To, From, Subject, and so forth—is called the *header.* Depending on your system, you may also see some cryptic lines with terms such as X-Mailer, received by, and id number. Most of the time, there's nothing of interest in this part of the header, so just skip over it for now.

Moving Forward

The contents, or text, of your message can be cut and pasted just like any other text document. If you and a classmate are working on a project together, your partner can write part of a paper and email it to you, and you can copy the text from your email message and paste it into your word processing program.

What if there are three partners in this project? One partner sends you a draft of the paper for you to review. You like it and want to send it on to your other partner. The **Forward** feature lets you send the message intact, so you don't have to cut and paste it into a new message window.

To forward a message, highlight it in the Inbox (top) and click the Forward icon. Enter the recipient's address in the "To" field of the message window. Note that the subject of the message is "Fwd:" followed by the subject of the original message. Use the text window to add your comments ahead of the original message.

A Chance to Reply

Email is not a one-way message system. Let's reply to the message you sent yourself by clicking on the **Reply** icon. What you see next depends on how you set up your Netscape 6 Preferences for Mail and Newsgroups, Message Composition. You were given the choice of quoting the original message within the text of your reply ("inline") or including the original message as an attachment. If you chose inline, you could also indicate if you wanted the quoted message to appear above or below any new text that you added for your reply. Let's assume that you chose "inline" and to have the quoted message appear above your new message.

Depending on which email program you're using, you'll see that each line in the quoted message is preceded by either a vertical bar or a right angle bracket. Note that the "From" and "To" fields have been filled in automatically and that the "Subject" field contains the original subject preceded by "Re." The vertical bar or > is used to indicate lines written by someone else (in this case, the message's original author). Why bother? Because this feature allows you to reply without retyping the parts of the message to which you're responding. Because your typing isn't quoted, your answers stand out from the original message.

A Discussion of Lists

There's no reason you can't use email to create a discussion group. You pose a question, for example, by sending an email message to everyone in the group. Somebody answers and sends the answer to everyone else on the list, and so on. At least that's the theory.

In practice, this is what often happens. As people join and leave the group, you and the rest of your group are consumed with updating your lists, adding new names and deleting old ones. As new people join, their addresses may not make it onto the lists of all the members of the group, so different participants get different messages. The work of administering the lists becomes worse than any value anyone can get out of the group, and so it quickly dissolves.

Generally, you're better off letting the computer handle discussion group administration. A *listserv* or *electronic mailing list* is a program for administering email to lists of subscribers. It automatically adds and deletes list members and handles the distribution of messages.

Thousands of mailing lists have already been formed by users with common interests. You may find mailing lists for celebrities, organizations, political interests, occupations, and hobbies. Your instructor may establish a mailing list for your course. For a list of searchable listservs, see www.liszt.com. Listservs come in several different flavors. Some are extremely active. You can receive as many as forty or more email messages a day. Other lists may send you a message a month. One-way lists, such as printed newsletters, do not distribute your reply to any other subscriber. Some lists distribute replies to everyone. These lists include mediated lists, in which an "editor" reviews each reply for suitability (relevance, tone, use of language) before distributing the message, and unmediated lists, in which each subscriber's response is automatically distributed to all the other subscribers with no restrictions except those dictated by decency and common sense, though these qualities may not always be obvious from reading the messages.

Get on a List Online

You join in the discussion by subscribing to a listserv, which is as straightforward as sending email. You need to know only two items: the name of the list and the address of the listserv program handling subscriptions.

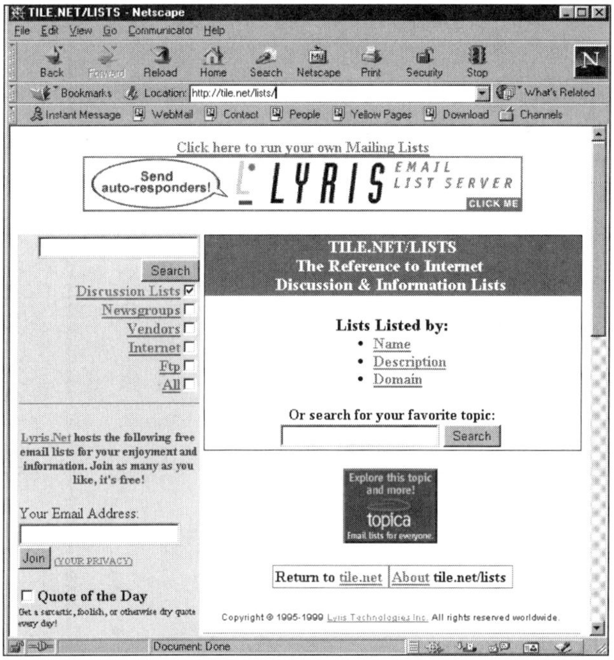

Tile.Net offers shortcuts to working your way through the Internet's maze of discussion lists.

To join a list, send a **Subscribe** message to the listserv administrative address (not necessarily the same as the listserv address, as the administrative address may serve a number of different lists). The message is usually as simple as "subscribe," the name of the list, and your name (your real name, not your username), all on one line. *And that's all.* This message will be read by a computer program that looks for these items only. At the very best, other comments in the message will be ignored; at the very worst, your entire message will be ignored. Within a few hours to a day after subscribing, the listserv will automatically send you a confirmation email message, including instructions for sending messages, finding out information about the list and its members, and canceling your subscription. Save this message for future reference. That way, if you do decide to leave the list, you won't have to circulate a message to the members asking how to unsubscribe, and you won't have to wade through fifty replies all relaying the same information you received when you joined.

Soon after your confirmation message appears in your mailbox, and depending on the activity level of the list, you'll begin receiving email messages. When you reply to a message, reply to the listserv address, not the address of the sender (unless you want your communication to remain private). The listserv program takes care of distributing your message listwide. Use the address in the "Reply To" field of the message. Most mail clients automatically use this address when you select the **Reply** command. Some may ask if you want to use the reply address (say yes). Some lists will send a copy of your reply to you so you know your message is online. Others don't send the author a copy, relying on your faith in the infallibility of computers.

You can cancel your subscription at any time. Simply send a message to the address you used to subscribe (which you'll find on that confirmation message you saved for reference), with "unsubscribe," followed on the same line by the name of the list. For example, to leave a list named "WRITER-L," you would send:

```
unsubscribe WRITER-L
```

Even if you receive messages for a short while afterwards, be patient—they will disappear.

Waste Not, Want Not

Listservs create an excellent forum for people with common interests to share their views; however, from the Internet standpoint, these lists are terribly wasteful. First of all, if there are a thousand subscribers to a list, every message must be copied a thousand times and distributed over the Internet. If there are forty replies a day, this one list creates forty thousand email messages. Ten such lists mean almost a half million messages, most of which are identical, flying around the Net.

Another wasteful aspect of listservs is the way in which messages are answered. The messages in your mailbox on any given day represent a combination of new topics and responses to previous messages. But where are these previous messages? If you saved them, they're in your email mailbox taking up disk space. If you haven't saved them, you have nothing to which to compare the response. What if a particular message touches off a chain of responses, with subscribers referring not only to the source message but to responses as well? It sounds like the only safe strategy is to save every message from the list, a suggestion as absurd as it is impractical.

What we really need is something closer to a bulletin board than a mailing list. On a bulletin board, messages are posted once. Similar notices wind up clustered together. Everyone comes to the same place to read or post messages.

And Now the News(group)

The Internet equivalent of the bulletin board is the Usenet newsgroup. Begun in 1979, today Usenet is a worldwide network of approximately 4,000 newsgroups. Usenet messages are copied only once for each ISP supporting the newsgroup. If there are a thousand students on your campus reading the same newsgroup message, there need only be one copy of the message stored on your school's computer.

Newsgroups are categorized by topics, with topics broken down nto subtopics and sub-subtopics. For example, you'll find newsgroups devoted to computers, hobbies, science, social issues, and "alternatives." Newsgroups in this last category cover a wide range of topics that may not appeal to the mainstream. Also in this category are beginning newsgroups.

Usenet names are amalgams of their topics and subtopics, separated by dots. If you were interested in a newsgroup dealing with, say, music, you might start with rec.music and move down to rec.music.radiohead, or rec.music.techno, and so forth. The naming scheme allows you to zero in on a topic of interest.

Getting into the News(group) Business

Most of the work of reading, responding to, and posting messages is handled by a news reader client program, accessible through both Netscape and Microsoft Internet Explorer. You can not only surf the Web and handle your mail via your browser, but also drop into your favorite newsgroups virtually all in one operation. For a list of newsgroups that can be searched by topic, see **http://www.liszt.com/news/.**

To reach newsgroups via Netscape 6, choose **Tasks** and then **Mail** to bring up the Mail window. Click on **File** and choose **Subscribe.** You will see a list of newsgroup categories and newsgroups. Click on the **Subscribe** column next to a newsgroup. A check mark will appear next to each newsgroup to which you subscribe. (Click **Unsubscribe** if you change your mind.) Now, click OK, and the subscribed newsgroups will be displayed in the Mail window. Double click on the one of current interest, and a list of messages posted will be displayed. For each message, you will see the subject, sender, and date. Click on a message to open its contents in a window.

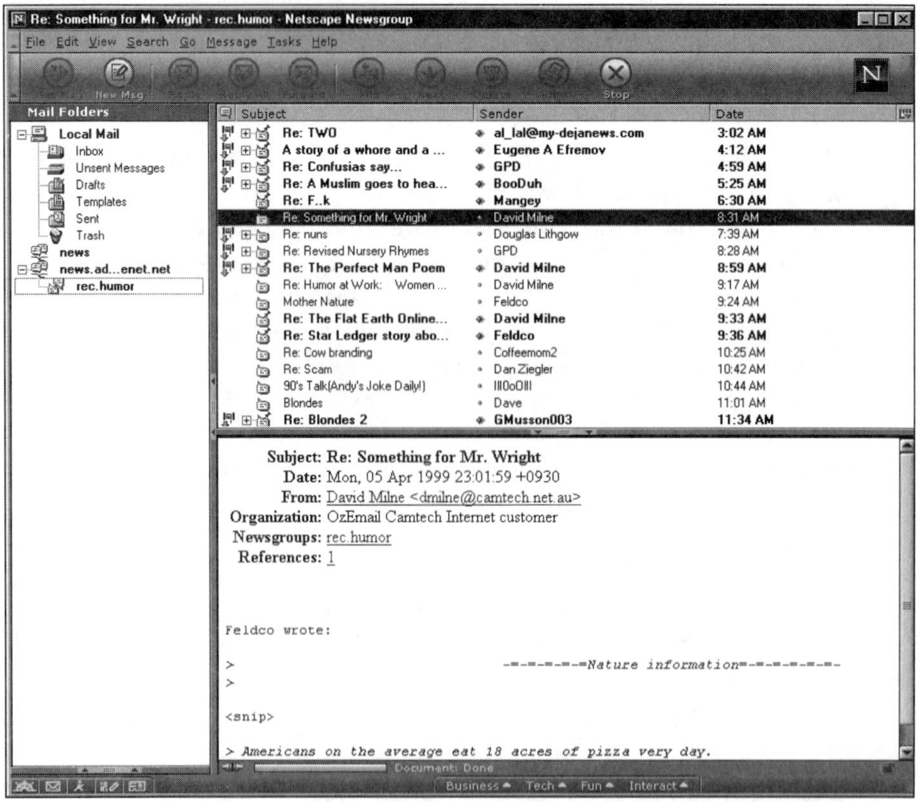

The top part of this figure shows a listing of posted messages. While not visible from this black and white reproduction, a red indicator in the Subject column marks unread messages. Double-clicking on a message opens its contents into a window shown in the bottom part of this figure. You can reply to this message via the Reply icon, or get the next message using the Next icon.

To reply to a message, highlight the message you want to answer and click the **Reply** button, then **Send.** To post a message on a new topic, select a newsgroup, click the **New Msg** button, write your message, and click on the Send button. Click on the **Get Msg** button to see your message within the newsgroup listing.

To reach newsgroups with Internet Explorer 5.5, pull up the **Tools** menu and select **Mail and News.** Choose **Add Newsgroups** to pull up a list from which you can choose to subscribe. Click on the desired newsgroup to see a list of messages posted.

Often, messages contain "Re:" in their subject lines, indicating a response to a previous message (the letters stand for "Regarding"). Many news readers maintain *threads* for you. Threads are chains of messages and all responses to that message. These readers give you the option to read messages chronologically or to read a message followed by its responses.

When you subscribe to a newsgroup, your news reader will also keep track of the messages you've read so that it can present you with the newest (unread) ones. While older messages are still available to you, this feature guarantees that you stay up-to-date without any record keeping on your part. Subscribing to a newsgroup is free, and the subscription information resides on your computer. Newsgroups have no way of knowing who their subscribers are, and the same caveat that applies to bookmarks applies to newsgroups. Information about your subscriptions resides physically on the personal computer you're using. If you switch computers, as in a lab, your subscription information and history of read messages are beyond your reach.

Welcome to the Internet, Miss Manners

While we're on the subject of Internet communication, here are some *netiquette* (net etiquette) tips.

Email Tips. When you send email to someone, even someone who knows you well, all they have to look at are your words—there's no body language attached. That means there's no smile, no twinkle in the eye, no raised eyebrow; and especially, there's no tone of voice. What you write is open to interpretation. You may understand the context of a remark, but will your reader?

If you have any doubts about how your message will be interpreted, you might want to tack an *emoticon* onto your message. An emoticon is a face created out of keyboard characters. For example, there's the happy Smiley :-) (you have to look at it sideways . . . the parenthesis is its mouth), the frowning Smiley :-((Frownie?), the winking Smiley ;-), and so forth. Smileys are the body language of the Internet. Use them to put remarks into context. "Great" in response to a friend's suggestion means you like the idea. "Great :-(" changes the meaning to one of disappointment or sarcasm. (Want a complete list of emoticons? Try using "emoticon" as a keyword for a Web search.)

Keep email messages on target. One of the benefits of email is its speed. Reading through lengthy messages leaves the reader wondering when you'll get to the point. Use short subject headings to indicate what the message is about.

Email's speed carries with it a certain responsibility. Its ease of use encourages quick responses, but quick doesn't necessarily mean thoughtful. Once you hit the **Send** icon, that message is gone. There's no recall button. Think before you write, lest you feel the wrath of the modern-day version of your parents' adage: Answer in haste, repent at leisure.

Listserv Tips. New listserv subscribers customarily wait a while before joining the discussion. After all, you're electronically strolling into a room full of strangers; it's only fair to see what topics are being discussed before wading in with your own opinions. Otherwise, you're like the bore at the party who elbows his way into a conversation with "But enough about you, let's talk about me." You'll also want to avoid the faux pas of posting a long missive on a topic that subscribers spent the preceding three weeks thrashing out.

Observe the list for a while. Understand its tone and feel, what topics are of interest to others and what areas are taboo. Also, look for personalities. Who's the most vociferous? Who writes very little but responds thoughtfully? Who's the most flexible? The most rigid?

Most of all, keep in mind that there are far more observers than participants. What you write may be read by 10 or 100 times more people than those whose names show up in the daily messages. Do not clutter up the list with "me, too" messages, or quote entire previous messages (only the part to which you're referring). Remember that messages arrive in the email box of subscribers and can fill it up.

Newsgroup Tips. Hang out for a while, or *lurk,* to familiarize yourself with the style, tone, and content of newsgroup messages. As you probably surmised from the names of the groups, their topics of discussion are quite narrow. One of the no-no's of newsgroups is posting messages on subjects outside the focus of the group. Posting off-topic messages, especially lengthy ones, is an excellent way to attract flaming.

A *flame* is a brutally debasing message from one user to another. Flames are designed to hurt and offend, and often the target of the flame feels compelled to respond in kind to protect his or her self-esteem. This leads to a *flame war,* as other users take sides and set flames of their own. If you find yourself the target of a flame, your best strategy is to ignore it. As with a campfire, if no one tends to the flames, they soon die out.

Keep your messages short and to the point. Many newsgroup visitors connect to the Internet via modems. Downloading a day's worth of long postings, especially uninteresting ones, is annoying and frustrating.

Similarly, don't post the same message to multiple, related newsgroups. This is called *cross posting,* and it's a peeve of Net citizens who check into these groups. If you've ever flipped the television from channel to channel during a commercial break only to encounter the same commercial (an advertising practice called *roadblocking*), you can imagine how annoying it is to drop in on several newsgroups only to find the same messages posted to each one.

With the huge potential audience newsgroups offer, you might think you've found an excellent medium for advertising goods or services. After all, posting a few messages appears analogous to running classified ads in newspapers, only here the cost is free. There's a name for these kinds of messages—*spam.* Spam is the junk mail of the Internet, and the practice of spamming is a surefire way to attract flames. The best advice for handling spam? Don't answer it. Not only does an answer encourage the spammer, but he or she will also undoubtedly put your email address on a list and sell it to other spammers, who will flood your online mailbox with their junk.

Above all, be considerate of others. Treat them the way you'd like to be treated. Do you enjoy having your grammar or word choices corrected in front of the whole world? Do you feel comfortable when someone calls you stupid in public? Do you appreciate having your religion, ethnicity, heritage, or gender belittled in front of an audience? Respect the rights and feelings of others, if not out of simple decency, then out of the sanctions your ISP may impose. Although you have every right to express an unpopular opinion or to take issue with the postings of others, most ISPs have regulations about the kinds of messages one can send via their facilities. Obscenities, threats, and spam may, at a minimum, result in your losing Internet access privileges.

Let's Chat

Virtual chatrooms let you communicate with others around the world in real time by typing on your keyboard. Unless moderated, chats tend to be rather chaotic, with comments going by fast and more than one conversation taking place at the same time!

When arriving in a chatroom, it's customary to say "hi" to whomever's there. Once you type a message, press Enter to send it. Since there may be a lag time between what you say and the answer, wait a few minutes. Do not type in all caps; this is SHOUTING. Describe your actions to make communication clearer (e.g., pounds on table for emphasis).

Types of chat programs include:

- *Web-based chat programs.* Web sites sometimes include a chatroom on a specific subject. Excite, AltaVista, and Yahoo all have free chatrooms. Look for a list of scheduled chats and topics.
- *Internet Relay Chat (IRC).* This method requires using special commands. An IRC server has chatrooms called "channels" where people talk, using nicknames. To use IRC, you need special software such as mIRC, a free program for the PC. You can download this program plus get instructions at the mIRC Homepage (www.geocities.com/~mirc).
- *ICQ*. ICQ ("I Seek You") began in 1997. ICQ networks contain lists of chatrooms. ICQ also lets you know when friends log on so that you can chat with them while still surfing the Internet. For this to work, both you and your friends must be using ICQ. See the official ICQ site at web.icq.com.

Netscape Instant Messenger is similar to chat in that communication occurs in real time. It is different in that messages are private, sent to an individual on a Buddy List that you create.

Virtual worlds, with either a social or educational function, also allow real-time chat. A *MUD (Multi-User Dimension)* or *MOO (Multi-user Object Oriented)* is a type of text-based virtual reality. It contains a narrative description of places, buildings, rooms, objects within rooms, and characters. You use special commands to chat with others, interact with objects, or create your own rooms and objects (with permission). Most MOOs or MUDs must be accessed through Telnet or a client program such as Tiny Fugue (tf.tcp.com/~hawkeye/tf/). Diversity University, an educational MOO, provides access through a Web Gateway located at http://moo.dumain.du.org:8000/, which makes it possible to see pictures.

Avatar virtual worlds contain two- or three-dimensional visual representations of a place. You choose a visual character called an "avatar" to represent yourself. You can chat with others or explore the world with special keys on your keyboard that allow you to walk, run, or fly! You must download special software to enter a virtual world. One example is ActiveWorlds at www.activeworlds.com. Try their free software, login as a visitor, and choose a world from the menu to visit.

Quick Check

Let's review the types of communication on the Internet:

- Email lets you send and receive letters electronically.
- A listserv lets you send email to a group of subscribers, and receive messages from anyone in that group.
- A newsgroup is like a bulletin board on which messages can be written and responded to by anyone at any time.
- Chat occurs in real time in a virtual chatroom.
- MUDs and MOOs are virtual text-based worlds. Avatar worlds have graphical representations of places and characters.

A Site of One's Own

Nowadays it's getting easier and easier for the average person to create his or her own Web pages. The advantages of having your own Web site are numerous: you can publish your papers and reports, post your resume, and even create photo albums of your family and friends. You need only three things to create a Web page: a file written in HTML (HyperText Markup Language), a server (a computer program that moves information on request) on which you can store your files, and a file transfer protocol (FTP) program to get your files onto the server.

Writing in HTML is very easy, and there are many resources on the Web that you can check out to learn the fundamentals. A good place to begin is *A Beginner's Guide to HTML* from the National Center for Supercomputing Applications (NCSA) at **http://www.ncsa.uiuc.edu/General/Internet/WWW/HTMLPrimer.html** and a *Web Authoring Reference* from the Web Design Group at **http://www.htmlhelp.com.**

But, you don't even have to know HTML to create Web pages. If you use the tools in Netscape or software such as Microsoft's FrontPage or Macromedia's Dreamweaver, you can design Web pages without learning any HTML at all (though knowing a bit about HTML really comes in handy!). With Netscape 6 choose **Tasks** and then **Composer** to use Netscape Composer, easy-to-use page creation software. If you have

Internet Explorer 5.5, choose **File,** then **Edit with MS FrontPage** to work on your web site.

Access to space on a server is offered by many colleges and universities as well as a number of commercial organizations. Internet Service Providers such as Earthlink and AOL also offer space on their servers for a fee. Companies such as Yahoo! (**http://geocities.yahoo.com/home/**) and Tripod (**http://www.tripod.lycos.com**) provide free server space as well as page builder software. You may have to put up with some advertisements thrown onto your site, but if you can't afford to buy server space, this is a good option. Remember: only when your files reside on a server can your Web pages be accessed through the Internet.

FTP client programs will help you transfer the HTML files you create on your personal computer to the server. You can download one of these programs, WS_FTP, at **http://www.ipswitch.com/pc_wsftp.html.** An evaluation copy is free for you to try for 30 days.

For more information on Web page creation, check out these sites:

- Introduction to HTML from Case Western Reserve University: **http://www.cwru.edu/help/introHTML/**
- HotWired, The Web Developer's Resource, from Webmonkey: **http://hotwired.lycos.com/webmonkey/**
- HTML Goodies by Dr. Joe Burns: **http://htmlgoodies.earthweb.com/**

Security Issues

How Not to Come Down with a Virus

Downloading files from the Internet allows less responsible Net citizens to unleash onto your computer viruses, worms, and Trojan horses, all dangerous programs that fool you into thinking they're doing one thing while they're actually erasing your hard disk or performing some other undesirable task. Protection is your responsibility.

One way to reduce the risk of contracting a virus is to download software from reliable sites. Corporations such as Microsoft and Apple take care to make sure downloadable software is virus free. So do most institutions that provide software downloads as a public service (such as the Stanford University archives of Macintosh software). Be especially careful with programs you find on someone's home page. If you're not sure about safe download sources, ask around in a newsgroup, talk to friends, or check with the information technology center on campus.

In addition, be careful about downloading suspicious-looking email attachments, especially from someone you don't know. Even if you know the person the message appears to be from, someone could have obtained their email address and used it to send you a virus. If the subject heading sounds strange, it's better to ask questions now than to download and be sorry later!

To protect your files, it's a good idea to buy and use a reliable virus program. Both Symantec and McAfee sell first-rate programs. Go to **http://www.symantec.com** to purchase Norton Antivirus software for either the PC or Mac. At **http://www.mcafee.com** you can get McAfee VirusScan for the PC or Dr. Solomon's Virex for the Mac. You can update these programs right from the Internet so they'll detect the most current viruses. Most of the time, these programs can disinfect files/documents on your hard drive that contain viruses. Don't forget to check files on your diskettes as well.

Crude as it may sound, downloading programs from the Internet without using a virus check is like having unprotected sex with a stranger. While downloading software may not be life-threatening, imagine the consequences if your entire hard disk, including all your course work and software, is totally obliterated. It won't leave you feeling very good.

Keeping Things to Yourself

The Internet is not private. Information you pass around the Internet is stored on, or passed along by, computers that are accessible to others. Your ISP may provide member directories that list all subscribers and their addresses. Your activities at a Web site can be tracked, including which pages you visited. Cookies, files left on your hard drive by certain sites, make it easy for advertisers to find out your interests.

Just as you take care to protect your wallet or purse while walking down a crowded street, it's also a good practice to exercise caution with information you'd like to keep (relatively) private. Although computer system administrators take great care to ensure the security of this information, no scheme is completely infallible. Here are some security tips:

- Exercise care when sending sensitive information such as credit card numbers, social security numbers, passwords, even telephone numbers and addresses in email. Your email message may pass through four or five computers en route to its destination, and at any of these points, it can be intercepted and read by someone other than the recipient.

- Send personal information over the Web only if the page is secure. Web browsers automatically encrypt information on secure pages, and the information can only be unscrambled at the Web site that created the secure page.

  In Netscape 6.0, an "s" is added to "http" to indicate a secure Web page. This indicates that a security system called SSL (Secure Sockets Layer) is in place. (The earlier Netscape 4 showed a closed padlock symbol.) From the menu, select **Tasks, Privacy and Security,** to bring up the Netscape Security Manager. Click on the **Information** tab to learn more about the security setting for the page (if available). Click on the **Applications** tab if you want Netscape to display a warning before leaving secure sites or sending unencrypted information.

  In Internet Explorer 5.5, an icon of a closed lock displayed on the bottom right of the browser indicates a secure site. When you are sending information, you may receive a warning message if the site is not secure. IE classifies Web pages as Trusted Sites, Restricted Sites, or Internet (all other sites). To change the default security levels, choose **Internet Options** from the **Tools** menu and then **Security.** For each classification type, choose the **Default** level for a visual view of the security setting (high, medium, or low). For example, Trusted Sites are listed as low security. Move the slider to change the level. For more detailed security information, choose the **Custom** level.Remember that any files you store on your ISP's computer are accessible to unscrupulous hackers. See if your ISP has a privacy policy, and find out what it says. Consider whether you really want to post a "member profile" with information about yourself.

- Protect your password. Many Web client programs, such as mail clients, maintain your password for you. That means anyone with physical access to your computer can read your email. With a few simple tools, someone can even steal your password. Never leave your password on a lab computer. (Make sure the **Remember Password** or **Save Password** box is unchecked in any application that asks for your password.) It helps to change your password often and use a combination of letters and numbers meaningful only to you.

- If shopping online, check for contact information such as a phone number. Ask others about the vendor's reputation. Do not click on links in email sent by advertisers (they're probably checking to see if your email address is active). Consider getting a separate email account from a free provider such as Excite or Onebox.com and using it for shopping.

- The contents of any message you post become public information, but in a newsgroup your email address also becomes public knowledge. Use common sense about posting information you or someone else expects to remain private. Many newsgroup postings are archived (stored for a long period of time) and can be searched by search engines.

Finally, remember that the Web in particular and the Internet in general are communications media with a far-reaching audience, and placing information on the Internet is tantamount to publishing it. Information can and will be read by people with different tastes and sensitivities. The Web tends to be self-censoring, so be prepared to handle feedback, both good and bad.

Using the Internet for Research: Critical Evaluation

Much of your time online will be spent on researching your chosen field. Typical research resources, such as journal articles, books, and other scholarly works, are reviewed by a panel of experts before being published. At the very least, any reputable publisher takes care to assure that the author is who he or she claims to be and that the work being published represents an informed point of view. When anyone can post anything in a Web site or to a newsgroup, the burden of assessing the relevance and accuracy of what you read falls to you. Rumors quickly grow into facts on the Internet simply because stories spread so rapidly that the "news" seems to be everywhere. Because the Internet leaves few tracks, in no time it's impossible to tell whether you are reading independent stories or the same story that's been around the world two or three times. Gathering information on the Internet may be quick, but verifying the quality of information requires a serious commitment.

Approach researching via the Internet with confidence, however, not trepidation. You'll find it an excellent workout for your critical evaluation skills. No matter what career you pursue, employers value an employee who can think critically and independently. Critical thinking is also the basis of problem solving, another ability highly valued. So, as you research your academic projects, be assured that you're simultaneously developing lifelong expertise.

The first tip for successful researching on the Internet is to always consider your source. A Web site's URL often alerts you to the sponsor of the site. Or, if your search takes you to a specific article within a site, go to the home page of the site and read about the sponsoring institution. CNN or MSNBC are established news organizations, and you can give the information you find at their sites the same weight you would give to their cablecasts. Likewise, major newspapers operate Web sites with articles reprinted from their daily editions or expanded stories written expressly for the Internet. On the other hand, if you're unfamiliar with the source or suspect its accuracy, treat the information the way you would any new data. Look for specifics—"66 percent of all voters" as opposed to "most voters"—and for information that can be verified, such as a cited report in another medium or information accessible through a Web site hosted by a credible sponsor.

Look for independent paths to the same information. This can involve careful use of search engines or visits to newsgroups with both similar and opposing viewpoints. Make sure that the "independent" information you find is truly independent. In newsgroups, don't discount the possibility of multiple postings, or that a posting in one group is nothing more than a quotation from a posting in another. Ways to verify independent paths include following sources (if any) back to their origins, contacting the person who posted a message and asking for clarification, or checking other media for verification.

In many cases, you can use your common sense to raise your comfort level about the soundness of the information. With both listservs and newsgroups, it's possible to lurk for a while to develop a feeling for the authors of various postings. Who seems the most authoritarian, and who seems to be "speaking" from emotion or bias? Who seems to know what he or she is talking about on a regular basis? Do these people cite their sources of information (a job or affiliation perhaps)? Do they have a history of thoughtful, insightful postings, or do their postings typically contain generalities, unjustifiable claims, or flames? On Web sites, where the information feels more anonymous, there are also clues you can use to test for authenticity. Verify who's hosting the Web site. If the host or domain name is unfamiliar to you, perhaps a search engine can help you locate more information. Measure the tone and style of the writing at the site. Does it seem consistent with the education level and knowledge base necessary to write intelligently about the subject?

When offering an unorthodox point of view, good authors supply facts, figures, and quotes to buttress their positions, expecting readers to be skeptical of their claims. Knowledgeable authors on the Internet follow these same commonsense guidelines. Be suspicious of authors who expect you to agree with their points of view simply because they've published them on the Internet. In one-on-one encounters, you frequently judge the authority and knowledge of the speaker using criteria you'd be hard-pressed to explain. Use your sense of intuition on the Internet, too.

As a researcher (and as a human being), the job of critical thinking requires a combination of healthy skepticism and rabid curiosity. Newsgroups and Web sites tend to focus narrowly on single issues (newsgroups more so than Web sites). Don't expect to find a torrent of opposing views on newsgroup postings; their very nature and reason for existence dampens free-ranging discussions. A newsgroup on *The X-Files* might argue about whether extraterrestrials exist, but not about whether the program is the premier television show on the air today. Such a discussion would run counter to the purposes of the newsgroup. Anyone posting such a message would be flamed, embarrassed, ignored, or otherwise driven away.

It's Okay to Be Critical

Your research responsibilities include searching for opposing views by visiting a variety of newsgroups and Web sites. It helps here to fall back on the familiar questions of journalism: who, what, when, where, and why.

Who else might speak knowledgeably on this subject? Enter that person's name into a search engine. You might be surprised to find whose work is represented on the Web. (For fun, one of the authors entered the name of a rock-and-roll New York radio disk jockey into MetaCrawler and was amazed to find several pages devoted to the DJ, including sound clips of broadcasts dating back to the 1960s, along with a history of his theme song.)

What event might shed more information on your topic? Is there a group or organization that represents your topic? Do they hold an annual conference? Are synopses of presentations posted on the sponsoring organization's Web site?

When do events happen? Annual meetings or seasonal occurrences can help you isolate newsgroup postings of interest.

Where might you find this information? If you're searching for information on wines, for example, check to see if major wine-producing regions, such as the Napa Valley in California or the Rhine Valley in Germany, sponsor Web sites. These may point you to organizations or information not found in other searches. Remember, Web search engines are fallible; they don't find every site you need.

Why is the information you're searching for important? The answer to this question can lead you to related fields. New drugs, for example, are important not only to victims of diseases but to drug companies and the Food and Drug Administration as well.

Approach assertions from a skeptic's point of view. See if they stand up to critical evaluation or if you're merely emotionally attached to them. Imagine "What if . . . ?" or "What about . . . ?" scenarios that may disprove or at least call into question what you're reading. Try following each assertion you pull from the Internet with the phrase "on the other hand. . . ." Because you can't leave the sentence hanging, you'll be forced to finish it, and this will help get you into the habit of critically examining information.

These are, of course, the same techniques critical thinkers have employed for centuries, only now you are equipped with more powerful search tools than past researchers may have ever imagined. In the time it took them to formulate questions, you can search dozens of potential information sources. You belong to the first generation of college students to enjoy both quantity and quality in your research, along with a wider perspective on issues and the ability to form opinions after reasoning from a much wider knowledge base.

Certainly, the potential exists for the Internet to grind out a generation of intellectual robots who regurgitate information from many sources. Technology has always had its good and bad aspects; however, computer communications technology provides us the potential to become some of the best-informed thinkers in the history of the world. Aided by this technology, we may become thinkers who are not only articulate, but confident that our opinions have been distilled from a range of views and processed by our own personalities, beliefs, and biases. This is one of the aspects of the Internet that makes this era such an exciting combination of humanism and technology.

Health Information on the Internet

Information relating to health, wellness, health care, and medicine abounds on the Internet. Web sites relating to any aspect of health are available with a few mouse clicks. What formerly took hours of searching for information from libraries can now be found in minutes. In former times, contacting colleagues to discuss important ideas required either a long distance phone call or a letter. Now, the Internet allows easy and immediate transmission of these ideas. Like-minded people from all over the world can now discuss ideas, pose questions, and receive new information at lightning speed—literally. The Internet has allowed health information to move to a new and very exciting level of distribution.

With the arrival of the Internet, people looking for health information can find it at every level. For the second grader who wants to learn about the differences between a fruit and a vegetable, it takes little time to find appropriate Web sites to gather this information. For the high school student who needs to write a report on the global situation of HIV and AIDS, information is readily available on the Internet. Similarly, for the scholarly researcher who is looking for information to support a theory on which to build a research study, the avenues are available on the Internet to find this type of information. The Internet has information relevant to every level of learning and there is almost no end to the quantity as well.

One of the premier locations for finding any type of health related information on the Internet is at a Web site called "Your Business, Your Health." This site can help you access nearly any type of health information that is online. This includes health news, health research, online health journals and magazines, and locations for doing health research. It also is an excellent starting place for finding information-specific health topics. The address for this Web site is: **http://www.siu.edu/departments/bushea/**

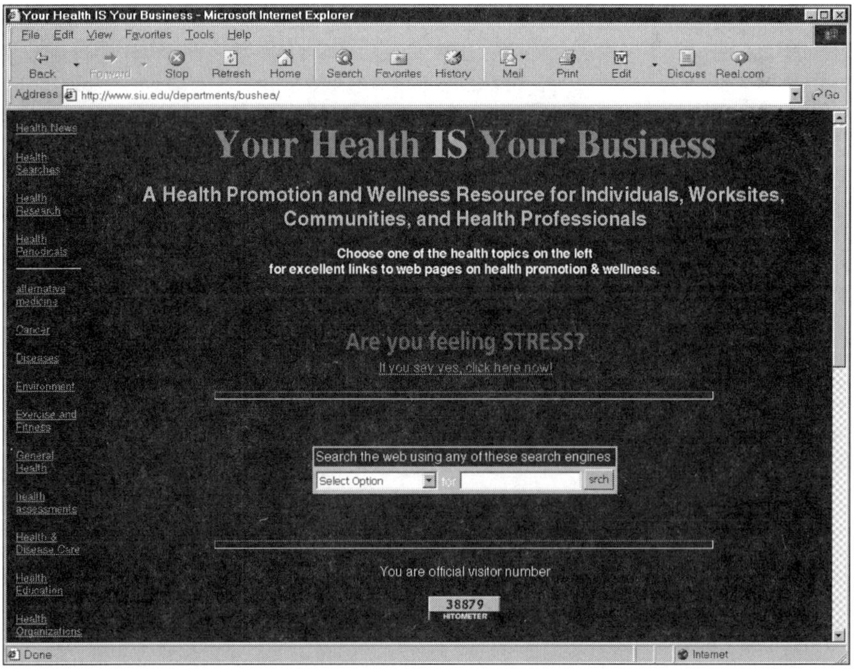

Using the Internet for Health Communication, Education, and Research

The Internet has quickly turned into an ocean of information for anyone who wants to know more about any aspect of health. A quick peek at a search engine such as Yahoo!, AltaVista or Lycos will quickly give us an idea of its immense size. For example, if we want to get information from the Lycos search engine (**http://www.lycos.com**) we can point our browser in that direction then click on the word "Health" in the Web Guides box. We immediately move to a page that lists topics such as: Fitness, Diseases, Alternatives, Women, Seniors, Health Care, Professionals, News, Diet/Nutrition, Men, Children and Medicine. Clicking on any of these topic areas will take us to long lists of related Web sites.

You may be asking yourself, "If there is so much information out there, where does a person begin when researching a subject or just wanting to know one particular idea?" For example, you may just want

part 1

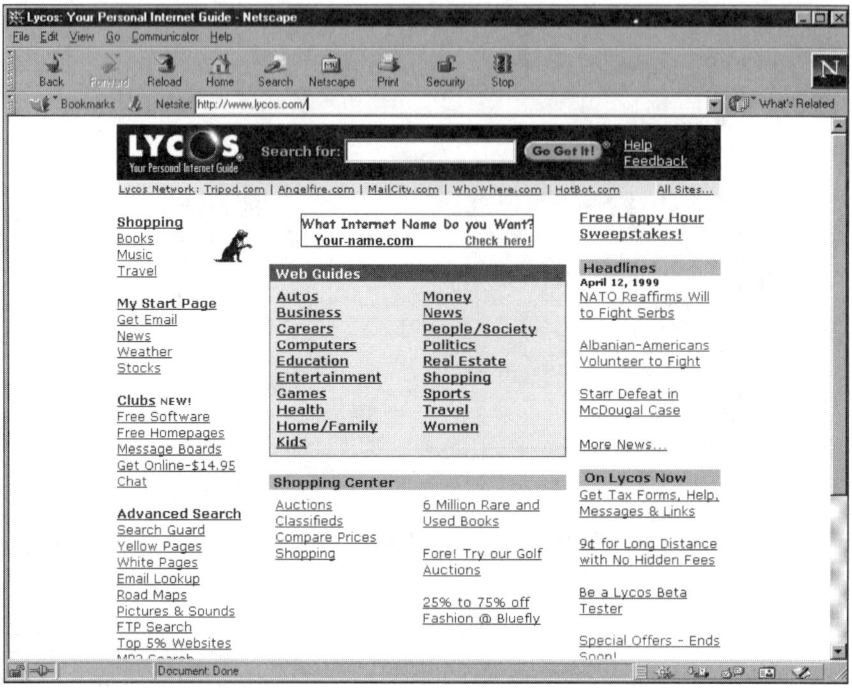

to know how many grams of fat are in the dinner you just ate at McDonald's. With a little bit of patience and following the steps and Internet addresses found in this book, you will be surprised how quickly you can find that for which you are looking.

Health topics on the information highway come from many different avenues. Many Web sites are designed for the sole purpose of giving out information. For example, a Web page dealing with weight control may tell you little more than data on foods and the various nutrients that are found in the foods. Other, more elaborate Web sites on weight control may have you fill out a questionnaire and then, based on your individual information, give you a printout of such information that is a bit more tailored to your needs. For example, it might let you know about the number of calories you need to consume daily to maintain, lose or gain weight. Considering your questionnaire, it may tell you how much exercise you ought to do during a typical week. It may give you pointers about what to look for on a food label to keep your intake of fats and sugars at a desirable level. Some Web sites are more interactive than others. The quality of the health related Web sites are as varied as the content.

Another aspect of the Internet, which makes it very appealing to those looking for health information, is the global nature of the Internet. People from all parts of the world can contribute to this sea of information as easily as can someone from North Carolina or Oregon. The rich diversity of the Internet brings some unique and interesting answers to many health questions. What makes this even more interesting is that many times, those who create these very interesting and unique Web pages place their email address somewhere on the page so you can immediately and easily contact them. Suppose you were reading someone's page on some type of alternative medicine for which you previously had no understanding. Perhaps after completing this information you still had some questions. Using the Internet and email you can easily set up a dialogue with that person by sending them a letter and asking them your specific questions.

Never before has it been so simple to learn all you could ever want to know on just about any topic relating to health. At times it can be frustrating when you consider the enormous number of choices. With some patience and practice, however, you are certainly going to enjoy the effectiveness and usefulness of the Internet at whatever level of researching you might find yourself.

Locating Addresses for Health Professionals

One of the amazing things of the Internet is the instant ability to find people and send letters to them. A perfect example of this occurs with health professionals. Imagine that you went to a health conference or watched television and you heard someone speak on a topic that very much interested you. After the conference was over, you wanted to contact that person to ask some questions that were not asked in the meeting. Using the Internet, you can quickly find the email address to that person and write him or her a letter. Finding someone's email address is not very difficult. To begin with, there are search engines that find email addresses (mentioned earlier). Additionally, many health educators and health professionals have their email addresses listed at specific locations. One of these places to find email addresses for health educators is located at: **http://131.230.221.136/hedir/directory/index.htm**

part 1

Simply click on one of the directories listed by job site, by name, or by state and country, and you will find the names of many health education professionals around the world.

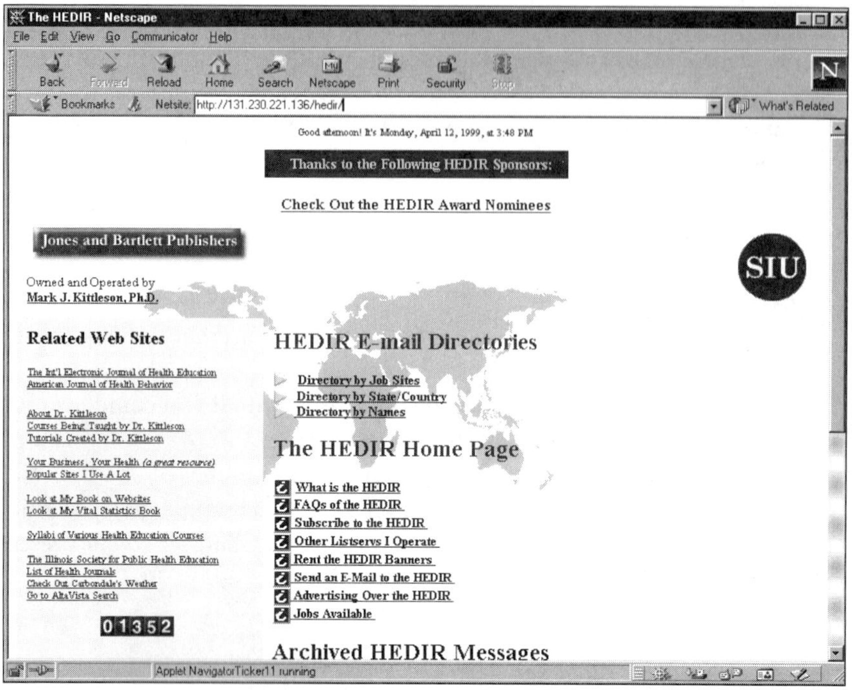

Locating a Newsgroup

Another way of gathering great health information is by connecting with a newsgroup. A newsgroup exists for nearly every aspect of health that you could imagine. About the only way to learn if a health related newsgroup might be interesting to you would be to check it out for yourself. Finding these newsgroups is not too difficult. You may type the words "health newsgroups" in your favorite search engine and see what you discover. After entering your request, the search engine will bring up many pages that list these health related newsgroups. One such page is titled "Liszt Newsgroups: health." Its newsgroups URL (Internet address) is: **http://www.liszt.com/news/search.cgi?word=health&an=all**

A long list of health related newsgroups appears. You may choose from any one of these that look particularly interesting. The titles in the listing usually give you an idea of the focus for each newsgroup. Some of the newsgroups to choose from at this point include the following: alt.hypnosis, alt.meditation, misc.health.infertility, misc.health.alternative, and own.health.herbs, to name a few.

part 1

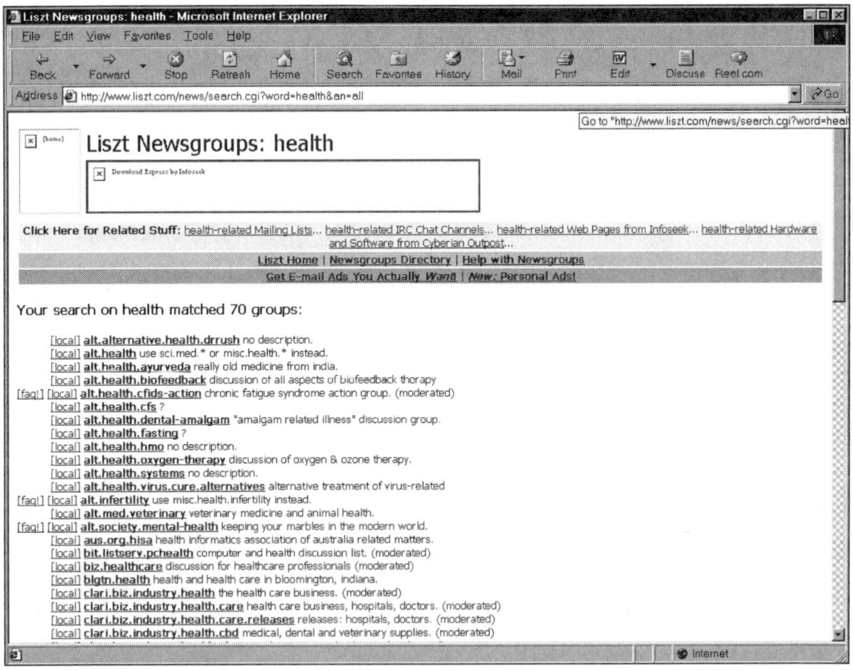

Finding a Health Mailing List

There is certainly no shortage of mailing lists for health. If you have never participated in a mailing list, doing so can seem intimidating. "Liszt: Mailing lists" (**http://www.liszt.com/select/Health/**) is an excellent "first stop" to locate a health mailing list that you may find interesting. It includes an enormous directory of mailing lists including such topic areas as: Allergy, Depression, Hospice, Exercise, Men's Health, Women's Health, and Weight Loss to name only a few. Once you arrive at this first page, simply click on one of the topics, follow the instructions, and very soon you are part of a mailing list.

Some mailing lists have several thousand people who read and contribute to the lists. With that many people, the possibility of a very large number of daily letters in your mailbox is high. At first it might seem exciting to receive that much email. If you subscribe to more than one of these mailing lists, you will be receiving an even larger number of email letters each day. It is wise to determine the amount of time you have to read your email. Follow the feel of the list for a month or two and see if

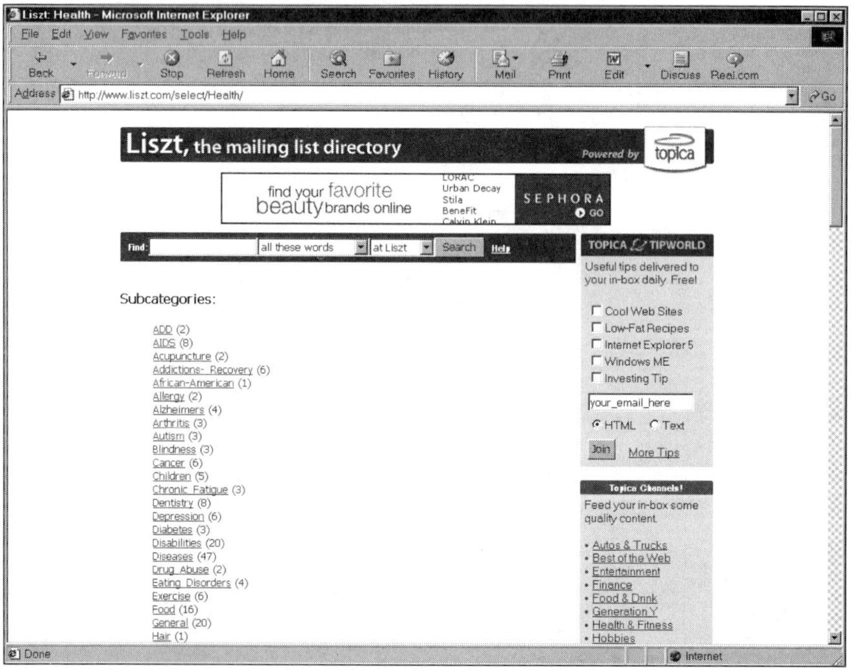

you want to remain subscribed to that list. Additionally, to avoid filling your mailbox, it is useful to set your browser to check your mailbox from time to time. Usually one check every hour or two is sufficient.

A Word to the Wise...

No longer is it a struggle to find what you need using the Internet. Be sure, however, to remember that there is no regulation as to what is produced on the Web. You do not have any way of determining the accuracy of information, so be careful. If you find information that is questionable or does not sound right, search elsewhere to get a second and third opinion. Use common sense when you are searching. If you are unsure about where to begin your search, refer to the Web sites in this manual as a guide. Happy surfing!

part 2

Internet Activities for Health

In this section you will find some activities that will help you use health related Internet Web sites in interesting and creative ways. Each of the activities will help you become more familiar with the Internet. They will also help you learn useful and unique ways to find excellent health information. These activities correspond with the health topic areas in the Address Book section of this text. You may find it helpful to refer back to these sections while doing the activities.

Health News

Something wonderful about the Internet is the speed with which information travels to and from all parts of the world. The research and developments that formerly took weeks and months to learn about are now available almost immediately. This activity will help you understand how this works.

First, go to the Health News page at the following URL:
http://weber.edu/hp/faculty/molpin/bushea/news.html

From here, click on any of the news sources listed. You will immediately go to recent health news stories. Try to see how many news articles or news clips you can find that have come out in the past week or two on the topic of heart disease. How many of those news stories discuss modes of treatment? How many describe ways to prevent heart disease? How many discuss risk factors for heart disease?

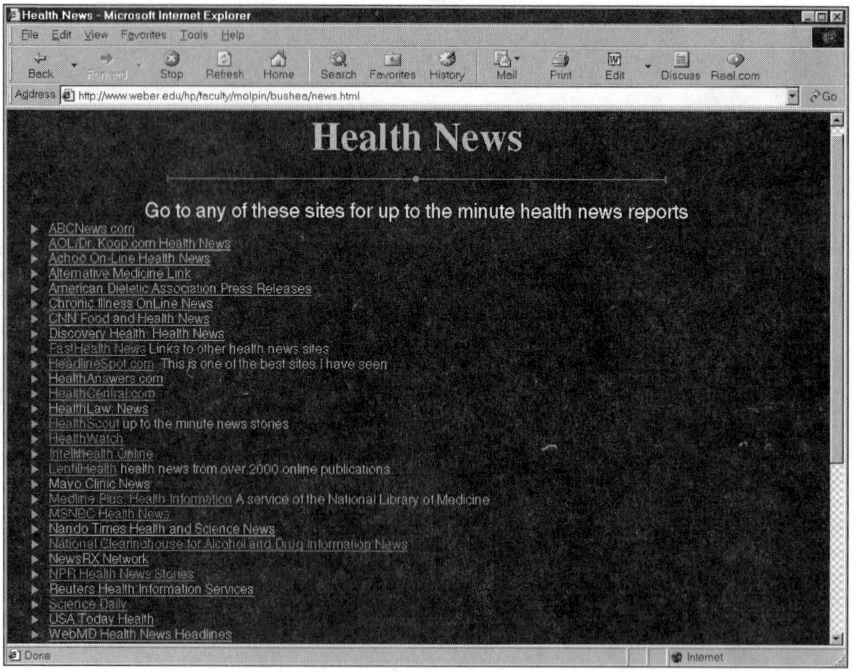

part 2

Do the same exercise for the following topics (or any others that come to mind):

- Cancer
- HIV/AIDS
- Diabetes

Health Related Searches

This exercise will help you to become more proficient at using the search engines to your advantage. You may begin this exercise by going to the following health search page: **http://weber.edu/hp/faculty/molpin/bushea/search.html**

Sexually transmitted diseases are a major health concern. Using the search engines on this page, find Web sites that give up-to-date information on the various types of sexually transmitted diseases that are common today. Look for current information on the following for each of the STDs:

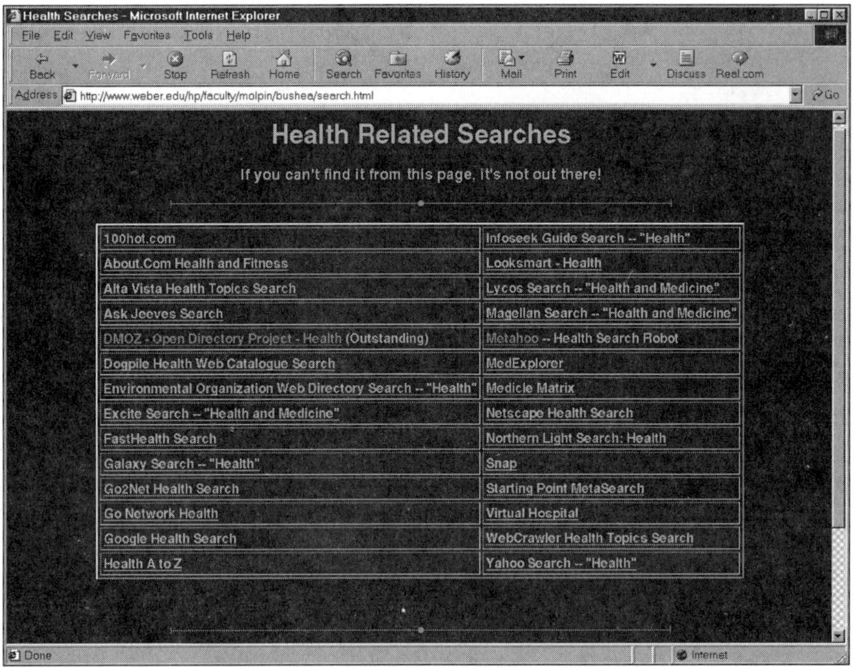

- Signs and symptoms
- Incubation periods of each
- Prevalence
- Treatment—which are curable, which aren't and how the curable are cured
- Prevention

For extra points, find pages with pictures of the various STDs, down load them and include them in your graphics folder on your computer to be used in your next report on sexually transmitted diseases.

Health Related Journals, Magazines, and Periodicals

The next time one of your teachers gives you an assignment to do a health report, try to draw primarily from these online periodicals listed in the section of Journals, Magazines, and Periodicals: **http://weber.edu/hp/faculty/molpin/bushea/journal.html**

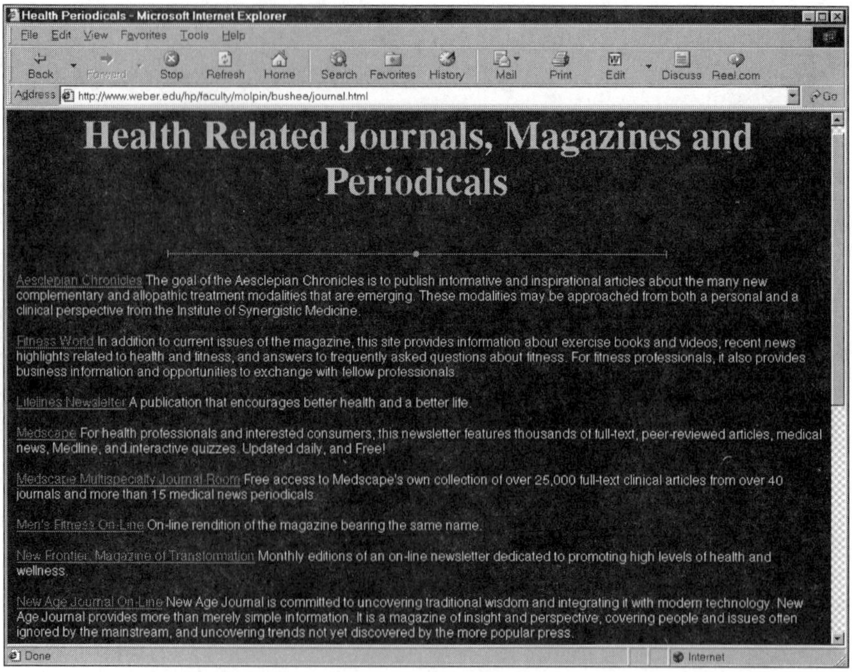

Do not use them exclusively but try to gather your information predominantly from these. See if the quality of the content of your paper is as good as the quality of those who use regular magazines, journals, and books to do theirs.

Health Research

Doing research on health topics can be unpleasant. The Internet has made the task of finding research easier. Although all research journals are not online, many journals' articles can be accessed from some of the research-based search engines. Medline is an example. To do a health research search, first go to this website: **http://weber.edu/hp/Faculty/molpin/bushea/research.html**

Next, click on **medline** to go to a medline search page. Once there, type a word or words in the text box that you want to research. Medline will bring up a list of related articles. You may choose one of these articles to see a complete abstract. If you have any questions, click the question mark in the upper right part of the Medline screen to improve your search.

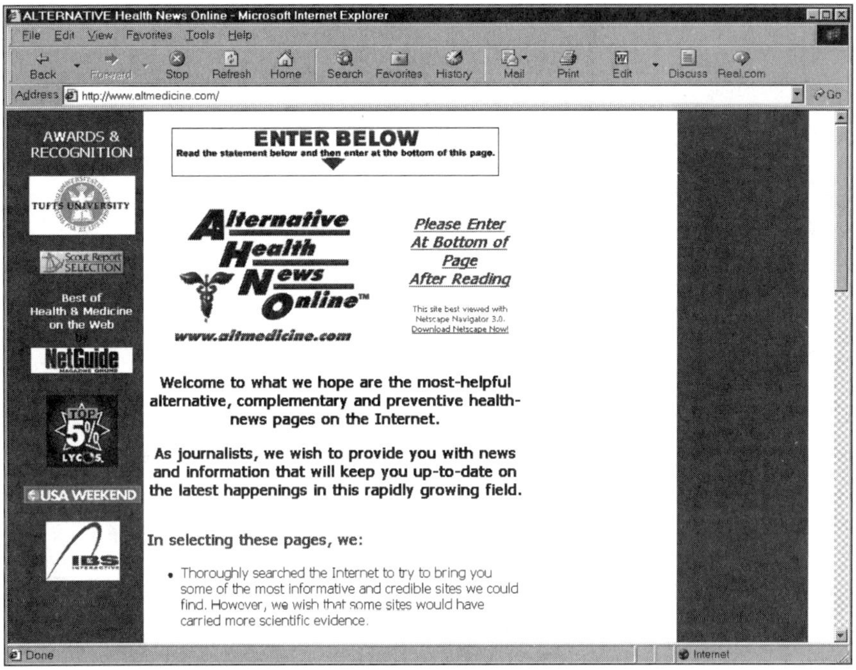

part 2

Alternative Medicine and Holistic Health

This exercise will help you gain a greater understanding of non-traditional or alternative forms of health and healing. In western medicine, we commonly treat headaches by taking an aspirin or some other type of pain reliever. However, there are other ways of treating the same problem without the use of drugs such as biofeedback, massage, acupressure or herbs. Go to the altmedicine.com web page at **http://www.altmedicine.com/**

Using this page as a beginning point, find several alternative methods of treating the following maladies:

Muscle pain

____

____

Arthritis

Constipation

Stress

Cancer

Heart Disease

Others

Cancer

This exercise will help you become more acquainted with cancer information. Try to find answers to the following questions using this marvelous cancer information page called CanSearch located at **http://www.cansearch.org/canserch/canserch.htm**

Which type of cancer is the most prevalent in our society?

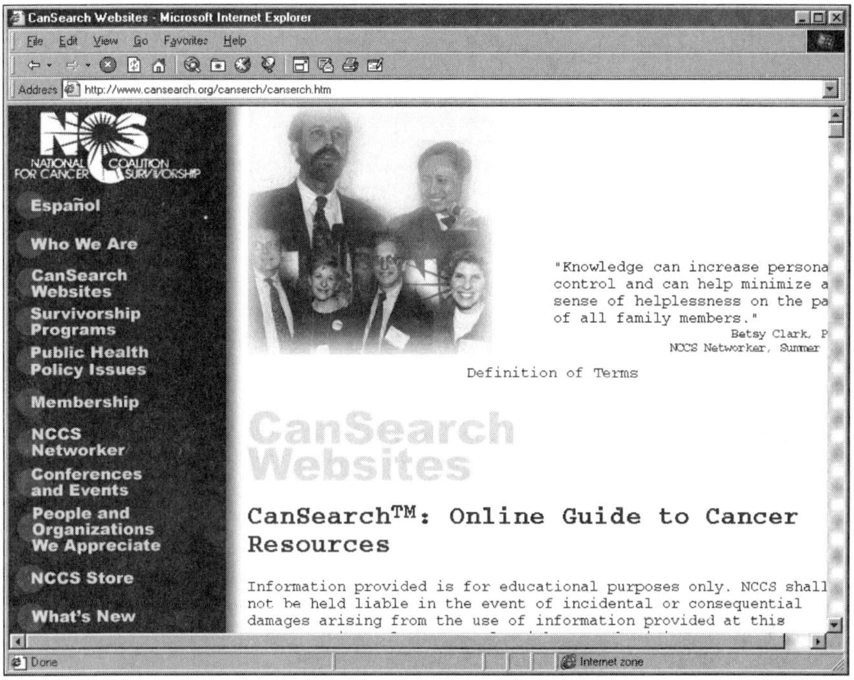

part 2

Which cancer has the greatest recovery rate?

Which type of cancer is usually the most painful?

Why is lung cancer such a dangerous form of cancer?

What are the best ways for women to decrease their risk of breast cancer?

What are the best ways for men to decrease their risk of prostate cancer?

What are the most common unconventional methods of cancer treatment?

Community Health

This exercise will help you gather current information on community health issues that face our society. The Centers for Disease Control (CDC) has an excellent Web site for all things relating to the health of our communities and society. Using the CDC's Web site: **http://www.cdc.gov/** Find the answers to the following questions:

Which states in the country have the highest rates for the following?

- Percentage of the population who exercise ____________
- Percentage who smoke ____________
- Percentage who are either overweight or obese ____________
- Number of AIDS cases by state ____________

Comparing men and women, describe the cancer incidence and cancer deaths by sites in the body (e.g., breast, colon, lung)

How healthy is the water we drink and air we breathe in different parts of the country?

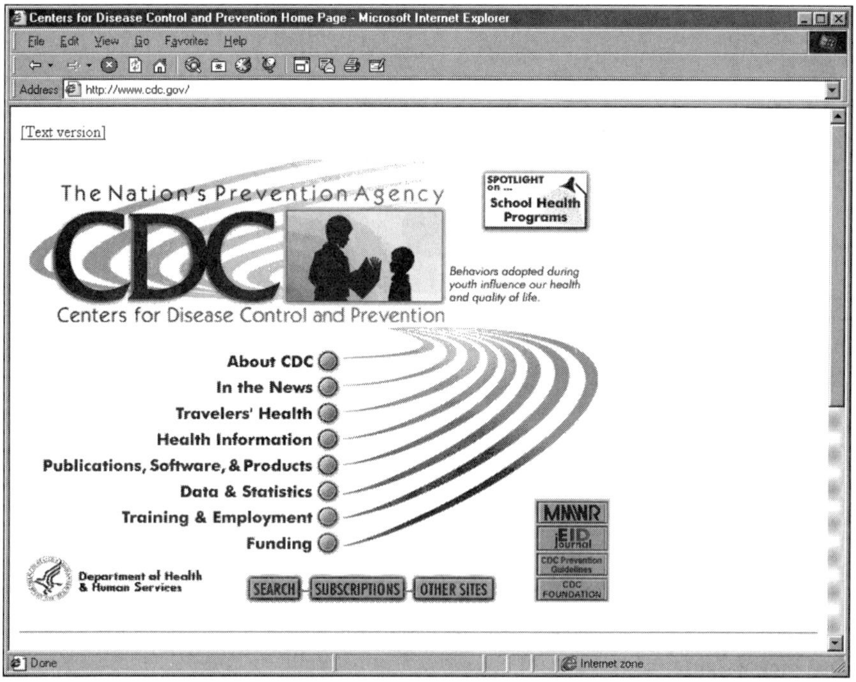

part 2

What are the leading causes of death in the U.S. for the following age groups?

- Infants ____________________
- Children ____________________
- Adolescents ____________________
- Young adults ____________________
- Adults ____________________
- Elderly ____________________

Diseases: Chronic and Acute

There are over 4,000 diseases known to exist in our society. Given the vast number and variety of diseases and illnesses, making sense of them can be quite a task. One Web site, The Karolinska Institute Library of Diseases and Disorders has put together a very impressive collection of most of the diseases of today. Go to this site by typing in the URL: **http://www.mic.ki.se/Diseases/index.html**

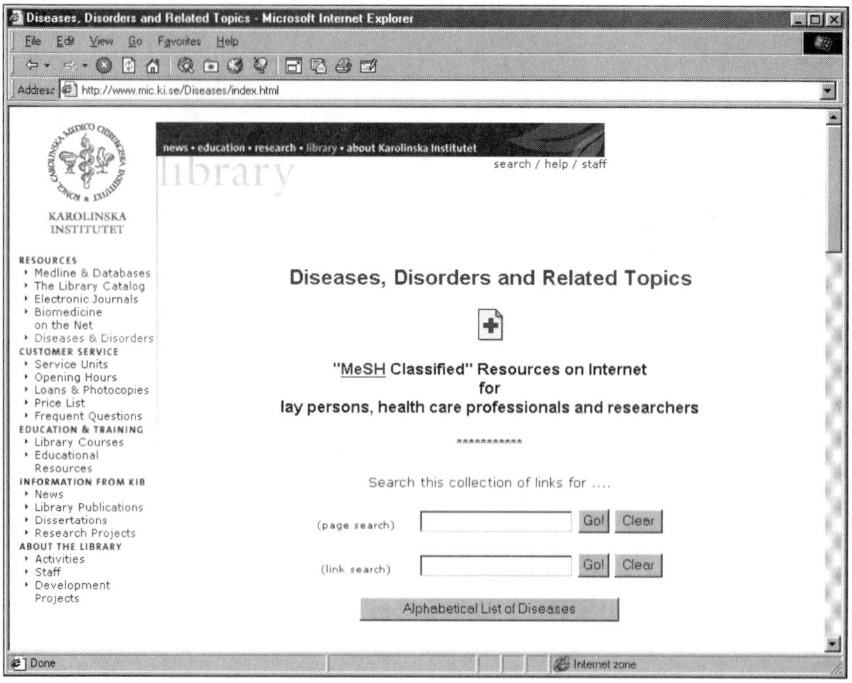

Browse this website to answer these questions (or any others that come to mind while you are searching.)

What are the common respiratory diseases in our society?

____

____

____

What are the common signs and symptoms of respiratory diseases?

____

____

____

What are the main causes for these types of diseases?

____

____

____

What treatments are available for respiratory diseases?

What are some common congenital diseases in our society?

What are causes and treatments for these?

This is an activity to learn more about how the immune system works. Using a metaphor, such as the sport of football, describe the immune system. Give the different parts of the immune system names that would apply in your metaphor. In the case of football, for example, the defensive line might be the T or B-lymphocytes. What part of the immune system would be the linebackers? What about the tight end, the defensive backs and the cornerbacks? Would the coaches play a role? How would the offensive positions on a football team represent other parts of the immune system? Be creative.

Environmental Health

Using the environmental health Web site, the Agency for Toxic Substances and Disease Registry, you will find the answers to these and many other questions relating to our environment. Go to this Web site by typing in this URL **http://www.atsdr.cdc.gov/**

What is the ozone layer?

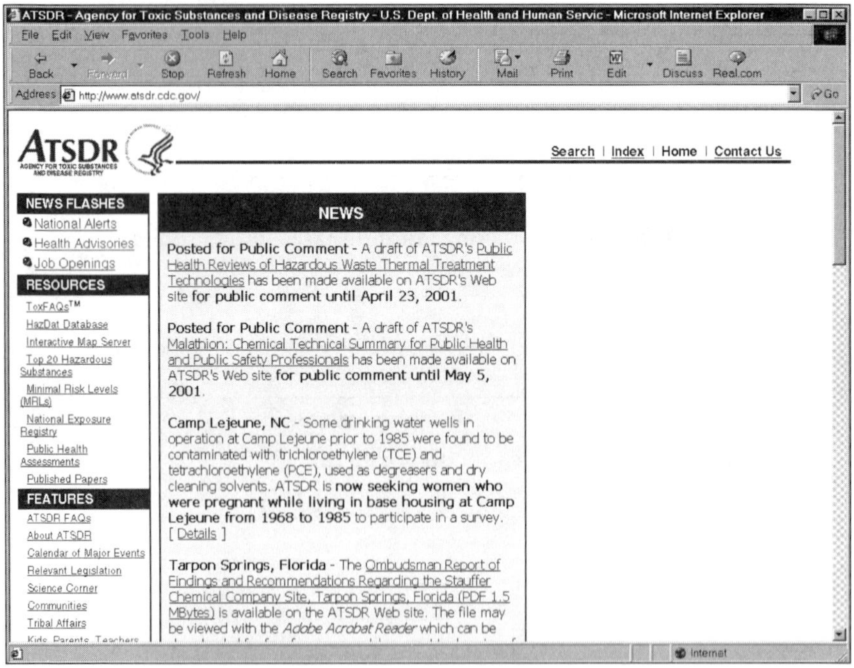

part 2

What is the current state of the ozone?

What are some common ways that we contaminate our water supply?

What does the Safe Drinking Water Act of 1974 say?

What are the most common sources of smog or air pollution in most cities?

What are some common health effects of smog or air pollution?

Who are the major polluters in your community?

What kinds of chemicals are they releasing?

Of these chemicals, which are the most dangerous?

How many pounds of the most dangerous chemicals are they releasing?

Where is your state listed in the Toxic Release Inventory ranking?

How does your county compare with others in your state for the release of these chemicals?

Exercise and Fitness

Few things we do can have more of a positive effect on our health than exercise. Attaining higher levels of activity and fitness is well known to be very beneficial. Go to HealthAtoZ at this URL: **http://www.healthatoz.com/atoz/fitness/index.asp** Find the answers to the following exercise questions:

What is your own aerobic exercise training zone based on your age?

What are the recommended guidelines for aerobic activity for you?

What is the best weight-training program for you to enhance your exercise/activity program?

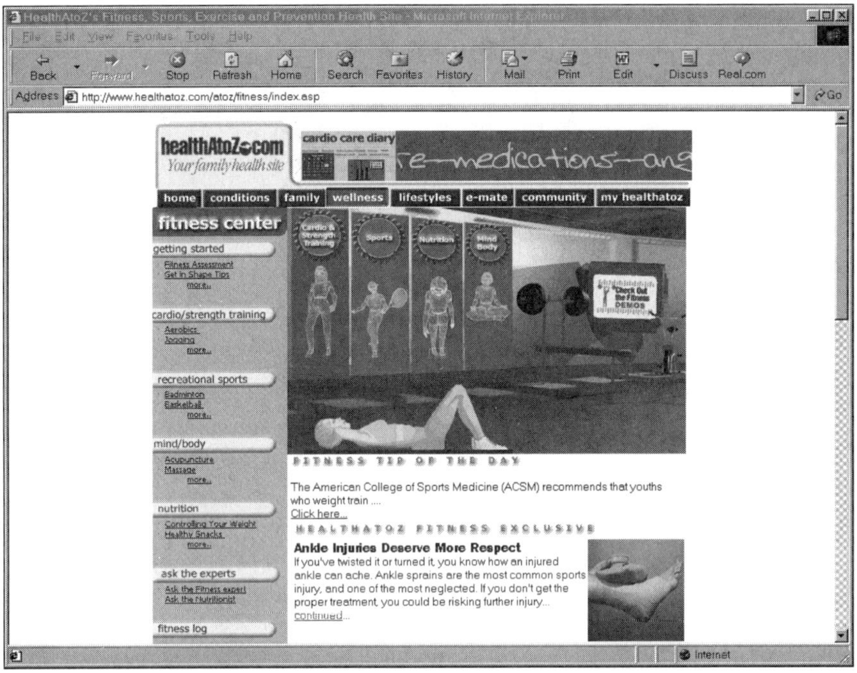

When is the best time to stretch out and what are some good stretches for you based on the types of activity you participate in?

____

____

____

General Health

The Web site, You First, at **http://www.youfirst.com/** contains a health risk appraisal. This health risk assessment includes all major factors relating to prevention and death: exercise, nutrition, smoking, alcohol use, weight, cholesterol, blood pressure, back pain, vehicle safety, stress, depression, and cancer. Once you've answered all appropriate questions, click on the "results" button to receive your personalized health report. Your health assessment will be calculated and a customized Web page containing your results will be built. Review your health assessment, and take note of how you can make each day count toward building

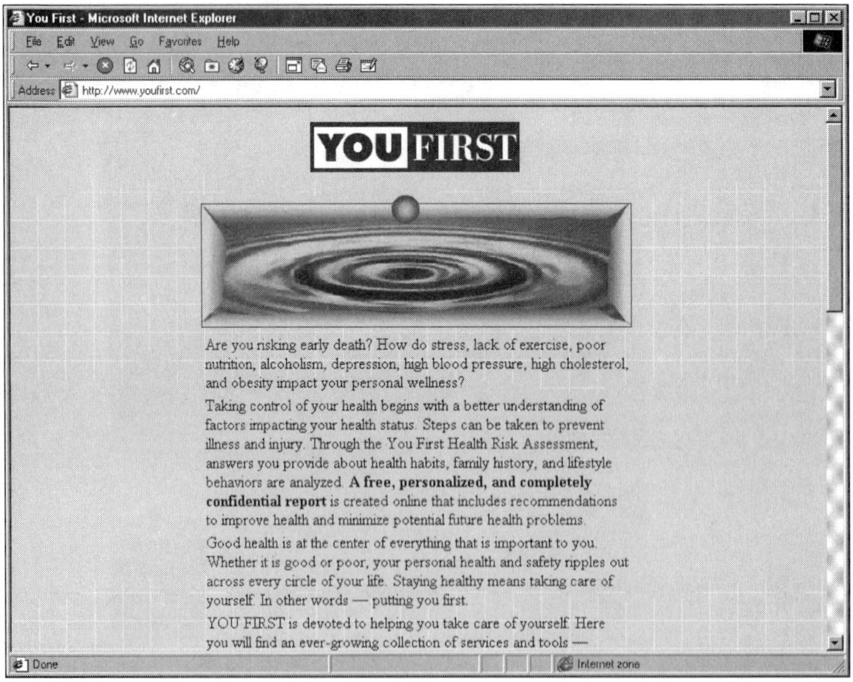

part 2

a healthier life. Based on the results of your health risk appraisal, how would you answer the following questions?

Are there current health conditions or habits that may lead to future health problems?

Are there actions you can take to avoid health problems?

In what ways can you improve and protect your health?

Global Health

Imagine you are on vacation to a South American Country. A large earthquake hits the town you are visiting. Buildings are destroyed. Hundreds of people are buried alive. There is no drinking water available and very little safe shelter for survivors. For this exercise, go to the website titled, "Global Health Council" at the following URL **http://www.globalhealth.org/**

See if you can find out which agencies would be most likely to be involved in the rescue and cleanup efforts and answer the following questions related to the disaster.

Who would lead the search for survivors?

____

____

____

Who would reestablish availability of food and drinking water?

____

____

____

Who would help with the cleanup efforts?

____

____

Who would be involved with sending in medical supplies, provide volunteers, and set up temporary shelters?

____

____

Government and Non-Government Health Resources and Databases

Here is an activity designed to help you find information on virtually any health related *organization* in this country and many others around the world. If you are unaware of where to begin your search, there are several Web sites that have started the process for you. The first one is **http://www.health.gov/nhic/** Once there, click on the words "Toll free numbers for health information." Immediately you will see an enormous list of health related organizations. Clicking on any of these will bring up an information page on that specific organization including how to contact them "toll free."

You will probably find what you are looking for by choosing the Yahoo! search for health associations. The address for this is **http://www.yahoo.com/Health/Organizations/**

With these two sites and a small investment of time, you can easily find information on just about any common, and some uncommon, health organizations that exist. You may also simply type in the words

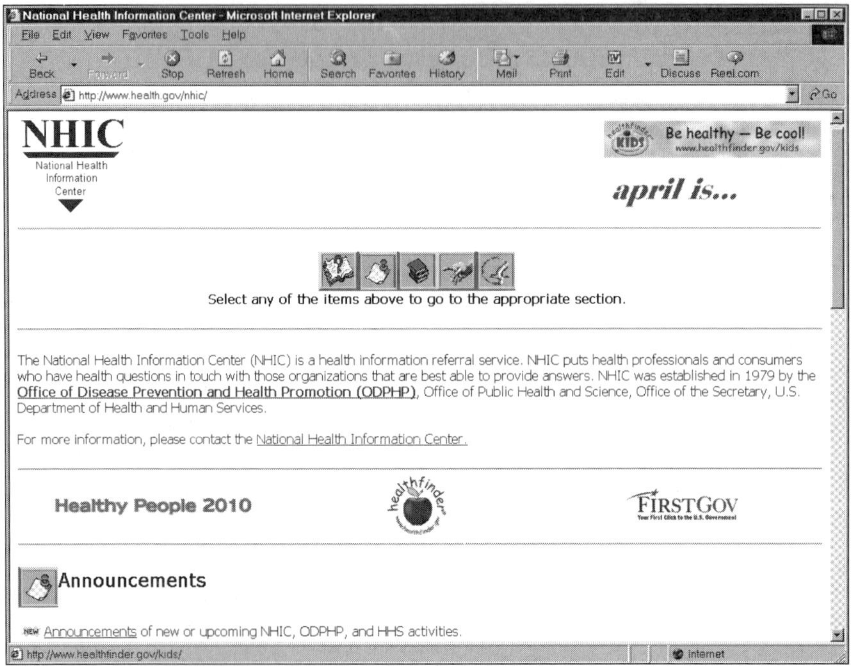

"health" and "organization" in the text box of any of your favorite search engines.

Health Education

Search through the Web site called Galaxy Health Directory at this URL: **http://health.galaxy.com/** Find three areas in community health that you are interested in. Then list several ways that health educators can play a key role to promote better health in these areas.

1. ______________________________

   1. ______________________________
   2. ______________________________
   3. ______________________________

part 2

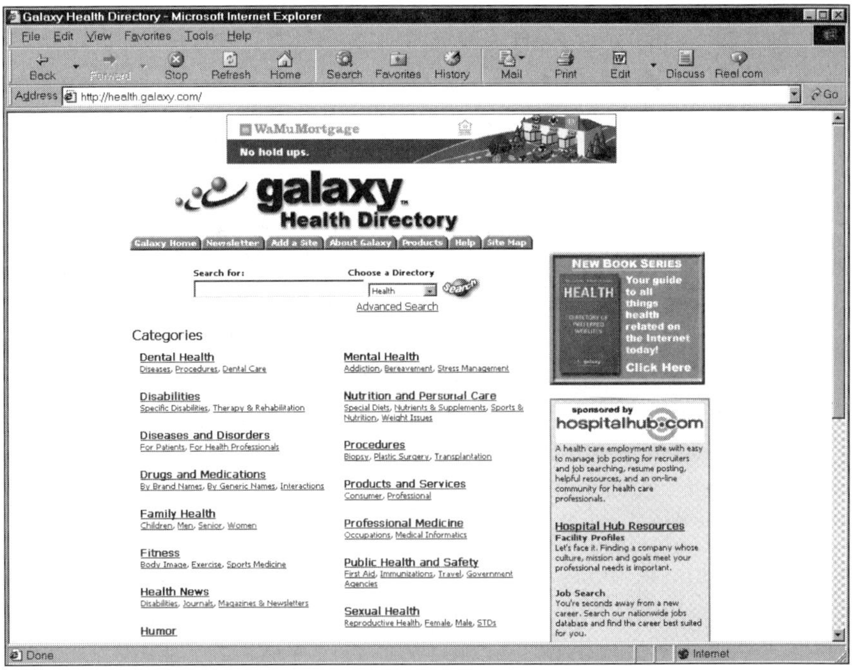

2. ______________________________
    1. ______________________________
    2. ______________________________
    3. ______________________________
3. ______________________________
    1. ______________________________
    2. ______________________________
    3. ______________________________

Health Psychology

A basic principle in health psychology is that of modeling. Modeling is one of the quickest ways of becoming very good at something. It involves finding someone else who has succeeded in doing that thing and doing the same things he or she did. This can be especially useful for beginning or intermediate health educators and health profession students. A nice activity designed to help you clarify where you want to go professionally follows a format something like this: (For this activity you will need a pen and a paper at first.)

1. Think of an area in health that interests you and write it down. (This may be quite broad such as fitness, or it may be more detailed such as a weight control specialist.)
2. Think of a setting that you would like to be working in once you are finished with your degree and write it down. (The majority of the health settings where health professionals work include the following: the worksite, the medical setting, the community, the school, or the university. There are many variations among these main settings.)
3. Think of how you might be working in that setting. What would you like your major roles to be? Write these down. (This might include something like managing a staff of aerobic instructors as part of a worksite health promotion program.)
4. Think of some ways you may be involved in assessing the needs of the setting. (How might you determine the types of health related

activities and programs that will be appropriate for this particular setting?)

5. Think of some ways you may evaluate the effectiveness of your program. (For example, if it is a weight loss program, what amount of weight will the people need to lose and over how much time will they have to keep the pounds off in order for you to feel like your program is successful?)

Now, having generated these thoughts in your mind, your next step is to find the people who are doing the same things and learn what they did to get there and why they are successful at doing what they do. This is where the Internet can be a very valuable tool. One excellent starting place in this search might be the following URL: **http://userwww.service.emory.edu/~cescoff/cam.html**

This page contains excellent information regarding the profession of health education. This includes professional certification, Health Education and Promotion Listservs or discussion groups, and State Health Addresses on the Internet. By subscribing to one of the listservs or accessing one of the professional organizations, you can quickly bring yourself into contact with many health professionals. You may also use any of your favorite search engines and type in the words "health" and "professional preparation." See what results come up and scroll through them. Once you find the person, there is usually a place where you can contact them using email, snail mail or even a phone call. Finding the experts and the successful people in your field is that easy.

Heart Health

This exercise will help you become more acquainted with the number one killer in our society—heart disease. Answer the following questions using the Heart Health Web site from the American Heart Association. The URL for this Web site is **http://www.americanheart.org/**

What are the various types of heart disease?

____

____

____

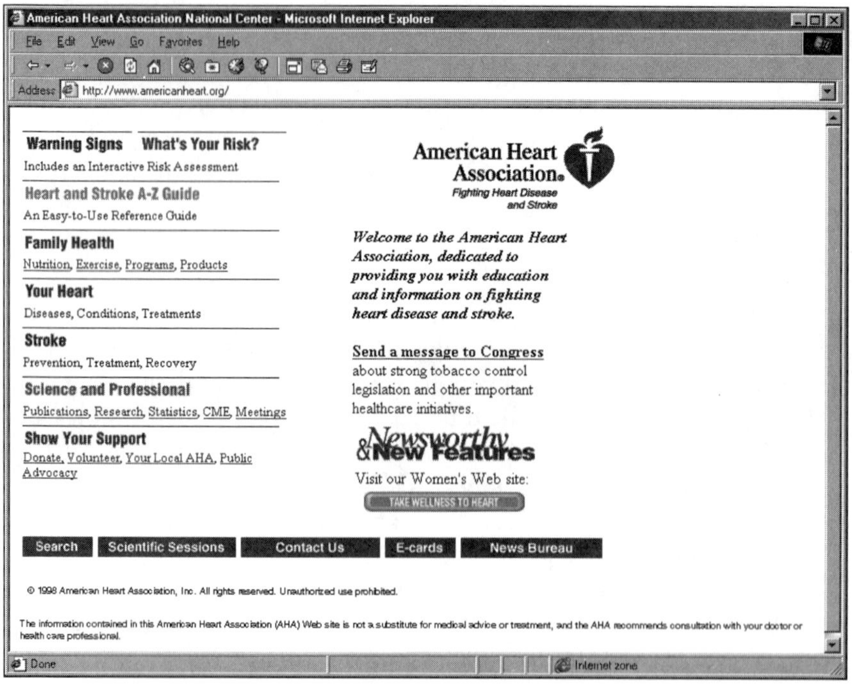

part 2

Can you find the average dollar costs of the various types of treatment currently available for heart disease?

What is angina pectoris?

In what ways does stress relate to heart disease?

How does a stroke differ from a heart attack?

___

___

___

Are there behavioral activities that can reduce one's risk of heart disease?

___

___

___

First Aid and Safety

Do you know what to do if someone begins bleeding? What if someone begins to have a pain in his or her chest and down his or her left side? How do you respond to someone who has a tick stuck in his or her leg or has swallowed some poison? Look through the Injury Prevention page

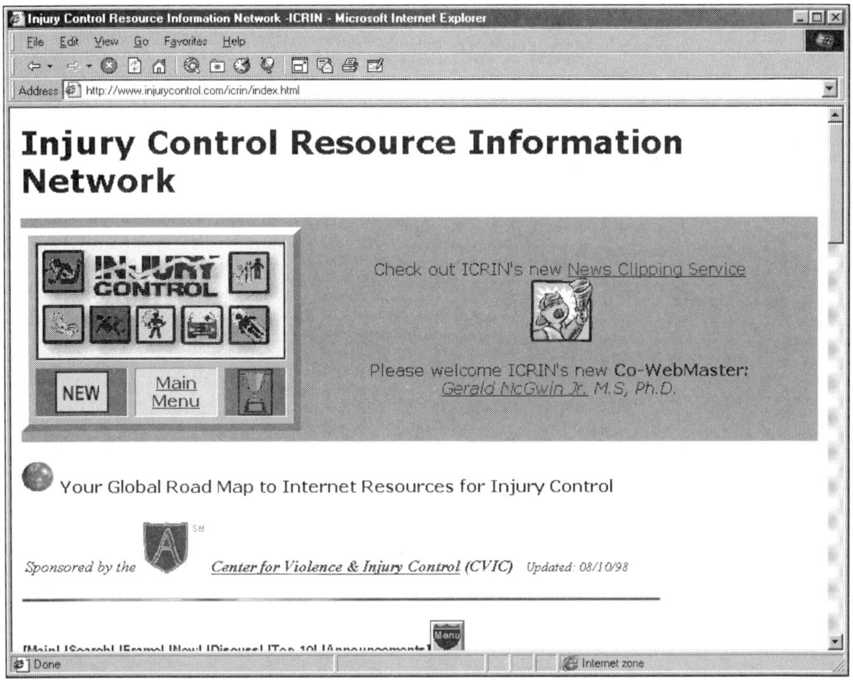

Injury Control Resource Information Network to find the answers to these and many other questions relating to first aid and injury prevention. The URL for this site is **http://www.injurycontrol.com/icrin/index.html**

Injuries

Begin this activity by going to the following website for the National Center for Injury Prevention and Control. Its URL is: **http://www.cdc.gov/ncipc/duip/duip.htm**

Choose any unintentional injury (drowning, scooter injuries, etc.). On the lines below discuss the prevalence amongst various groups (male, female, age group, etc.). Describe the costs to society economically and any other information that may seem appropriate and interesting. Next, look through the information on that cause of death or injury and describe what, if anything is actively being done to alleviate this concern.

____

____

____

____

____

____

Nutrition and Weight Control

For this exercise, first think of your favorite dinner at your favorite fast food restaurant. Write down each item on a piece of paper (For example: a Wendy's double hamburger with cheese, Biggie fries, large Frosty, and a cookie). Using the Fast Food Finder Web site at **http://www.olen.com/food/**, see if you can figure out the answers to the following questions.

What is the total number of calories for the meal? ____________

What is the total number of fat calories for the meal? ____________

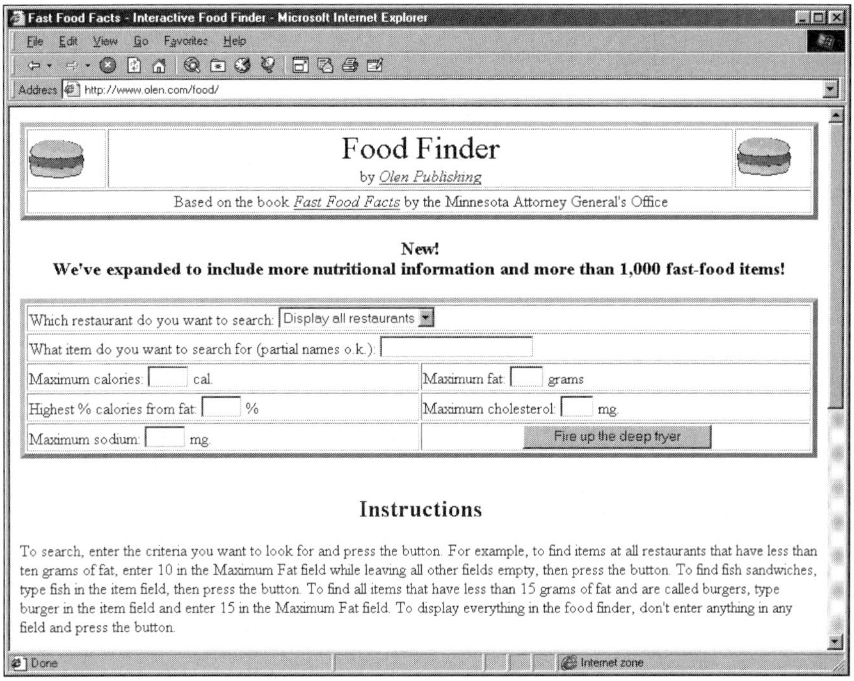

part 2

What is the total number of saturated fat calories? ___________

What is the percentage of fat calories for the meal? ___________

What is the percentage of saturated fat calories? ___________

What is the total number of simple sugar (simple carbohydrate) calories? ___________

How does your meal stack up with current recommendations for good nutrition?

____

____

Public Health

Here is a little activity that will thoroughly amaze you. I promise. First type in the following Web site in your browser's URL window

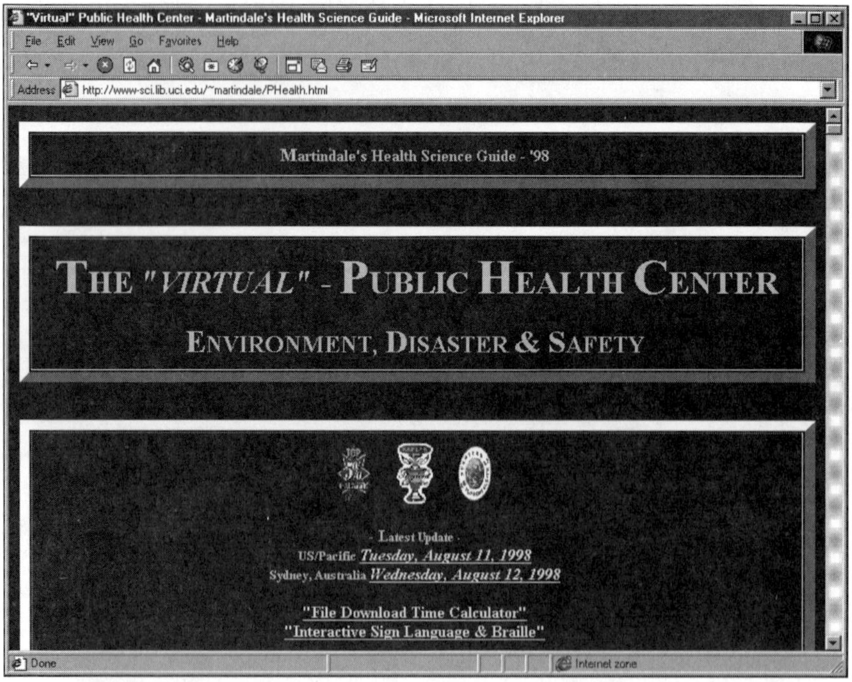

part 2

http://www-sci.lib.uci.edu/~martindale/PHealth.html This Web site is called *The Virtual Public Health Center.* You will find that you can easily spend a few minutes or a few hours at this one location. Just look through all the variety of activities and information relating not only to public health, but also to a host of other subjects that are health related. This is one of the finest Web sites out there. Stop in for a visit. You will not be disappointed!

Self-Help and Self-Care

You have a relative who suffers from chemical hypersensitivity or environmental illness. Using Health World OnLine at **http://www.healthy.net/**, find at least three different support groups or agencies where she can go for help.

1. ______________________________
2. ______________________________
3. ______________________________

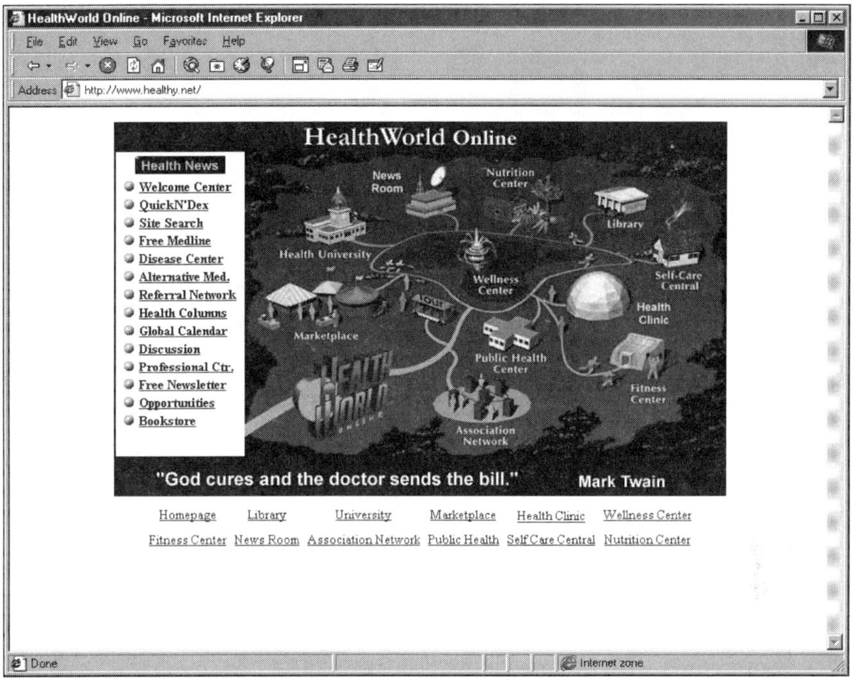

part 2

Stress Management

Stress affects us all, but not in the same ways. For this reason, we must have many ways to manage and reduce our stress before it adversely affects us. Experts say that sixty to ninety percent of hospital admissions have a stress component. For this activity, go to the stress management Web site titled "Mind Tools." The URL for this wonderful Web site is: **http://www.mindtools.com/smphyrel.html.**

Using the information from this page and the links to other excellent stress management places, list 5 ways that you could effectively reduce the amount of stress in your life.

1. ____________________
2. ____________________
3. ____________________
4. ____________________
5. ____________________

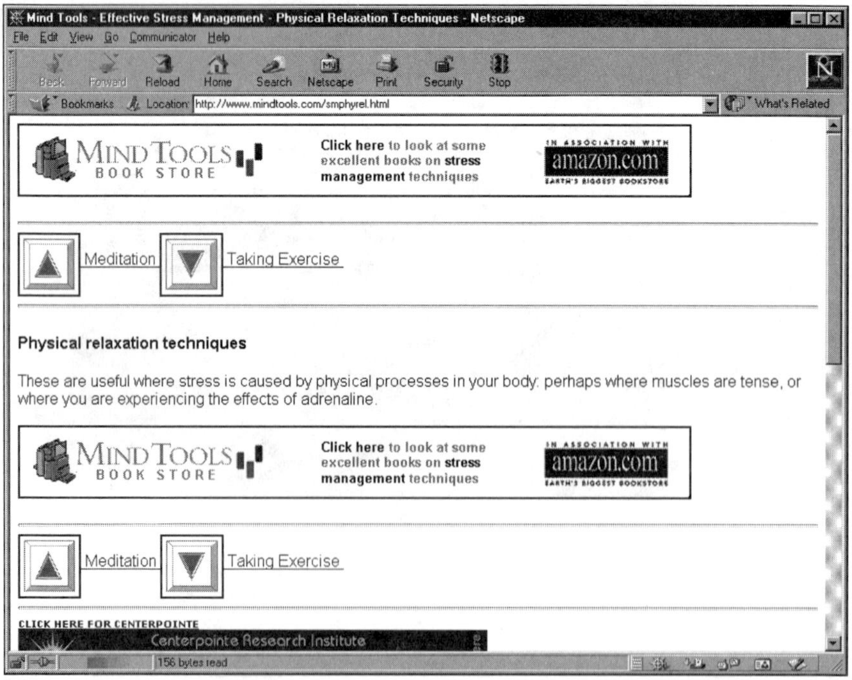

part 2

Tobacco, Alcohol, and Drug Use

Go to the National Clearinghouse Prevline at **http://www.health.org/.** Click on Alcohol and Drug Facts on the left side of the page. Using this information find out how many drinks it takes for you to reach certain blood alcohol levels. How much alcohol constitutes one drink? What are the effects on your driving and decision making abilities after two drinks? Imagine (or you may not have to) that you have a friend who may have a problem with alcohol or drugs. Proceed to: **http://www.health.org/govpubs/rpo884/**

Go over the checklist provided, making note of the areas that pertain to your friend. Then find several referrals to help your friend with this problem.

1. ______________________________

2. ______________________________

3. ______________________________

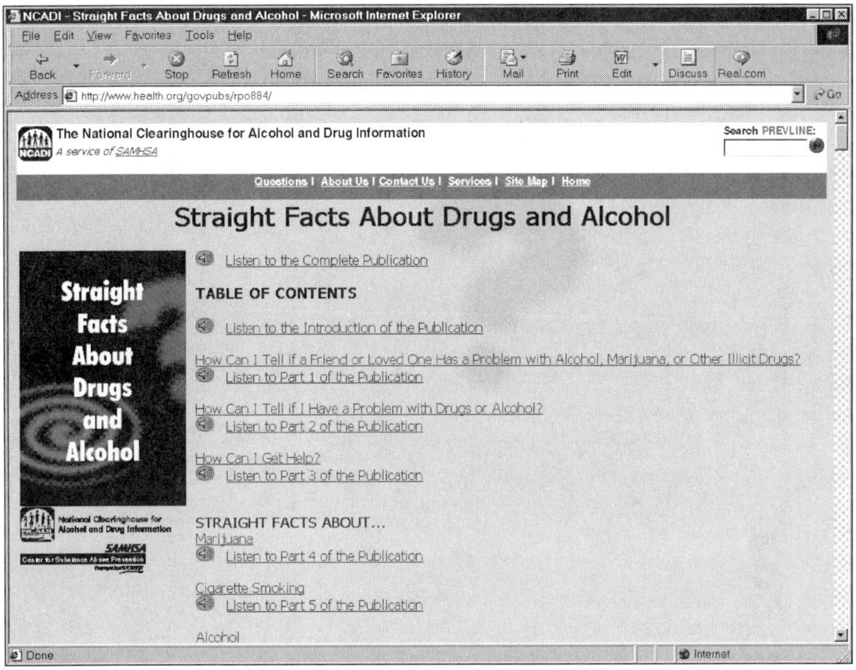

part 2

Wellness and Optimum Health

Based on the information found in the Wellness and Optimum Health resource sites at **http://www.weber.edu/hp/faculty/molpin/bushea/wellness.html,** create your own health newsletter.

Design the letter around your specific interests in health. You may want to include local community health information, pictures, and health articles. After creating the newsletter, print several copies and distribute them to your friends, family, or coworkers. You may even want to distribute them to community members in your area.

Women's Health

You have a friend who has just discovered she is pregnant. She is interested in learning about her childbirth options. Help her identify her options using the Website titled the National Women's Health

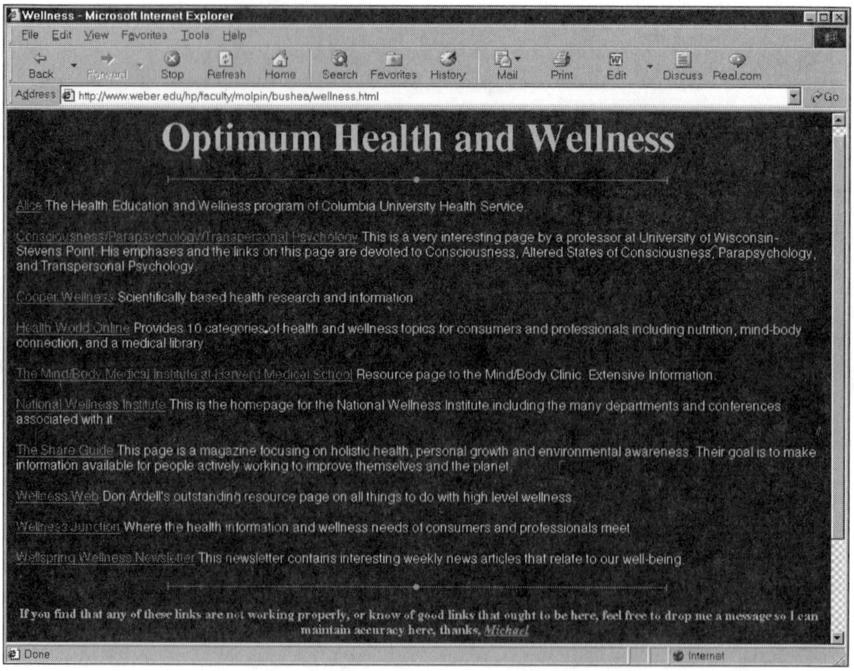

part
2

Information Center at **http://www.4woman.gov/** Also help her answer the following:

1. What are the differences between midwives and obstetricians?

____

____

2. What should she know about delivering in a hospital, a birthing center, or at home?

____

____

____

3. What other options does she have?

____

____

____

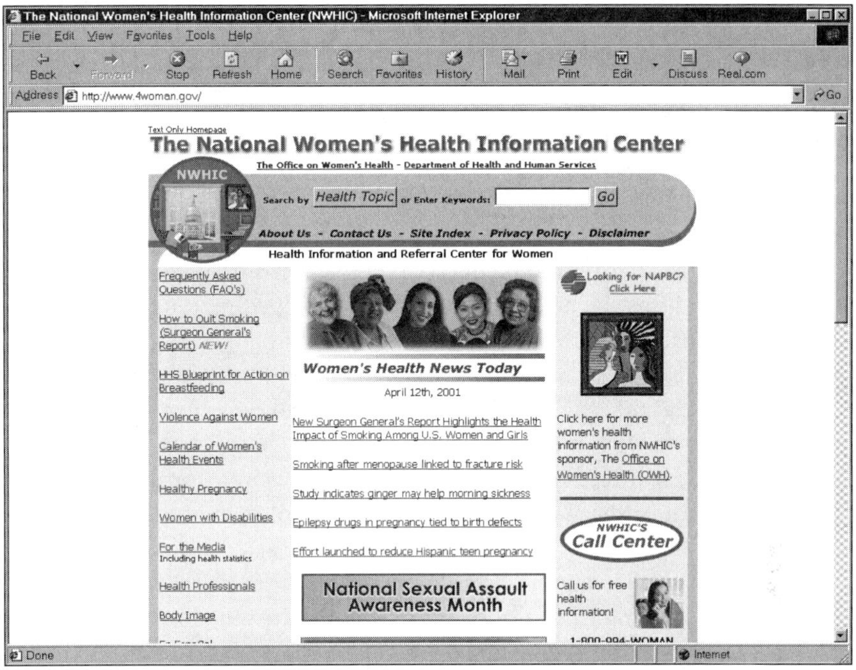

4. Should she exercise during pregnancy?

5. What are common complications resulting from pregnancy?

6. What routine tests will she be given and what do the results mean?

7. What are five more sources, support groups, or agencies she can contact for further information?

Health Related Web Sites on the Internet

This section is filled with Web sites related to all aspects of health. Each site is listed first with the URL (Universal Resource Locator) which is the Internet address. These addresses must be typed in your browser's URL text box exactly as they are shown. If any part of the URL is missing, you will not arrive where you want to go. The second part of the listings below is the title for each Web site. This is followed by a short description of what is to be found at the particular Web site.

One thing is sure about the Internet—it is in a constant state of change. All of the Web sites listed in this book were functioning at the time of publication. The Web sites that were selected for this book are ones that have been quite stable over the past few years.

part 2

Every listing in this book can also be accessed from the following health promotion Web page:

`http://weber.edu/hp/faculty/molpin/bushea/index.html`

You can save yourself some time by creating a "bookmark" to this page using your Web browser.

The Web sites that follow are categorized first by the following topics: Health News, Health Related Internet Searches, Health Related Journals, Magazines, and Periodicals, and Health Research and Evaluation. These are followed by the following health content areas: Alternative Medicine, Cancer, Community Health Education, Diseases, Environment, Exercise and Fitness, General Health, Government Health Resources, Health & Disease Care, Health Education, Health Organizations, Health Promotion, Health Psychology, Heart Health, Nutrition, Public Health, Safety & Injury Prevention, Self-Care, Stress Management, Tobacco, Alcohol & Drugs, Violence, Weight Control, Wellness, and Women's Health.

Health News

ABCNews.com

`http://abcnews.go.com/sections/Living/`

Health News from ABC News.

Achoo On-Line Health News

http://www.achoo.com/news/default.asp

Achoo News & Press is a comprehensive, Web-based healthcare news service for general public. Hundreds of timely healthcare headlines are categorized into hundreds of news topics.

AOL/Dr. Koop.com Health News

http://aol.drkoop.com/news/

AOL and Dr Koop team up on this website and provide the latest health news stories.

Alternative Medicine News

http://www.all-natural.com/news.html

Some of the most helpful alternative, complementary, and preventive health-news pages on the Internet can be found here.

American Dietetic Association Press Releases

http://www.eatright.org/news/

Find up-to-date news stories related to nutrition recently released by the ADA.

Chronic Illness OnLine News

http://www.chronicillnet.org/online/

Chronic Illness Online News has news stories relating to chronic illnesses and disease.

CNN Food and Health News

http://cnn.com/HEALTH/index.html

Find recent news regarding nutrition and health from science from CNN.

Discovery Health: Health News

http://health.discovery.com/

Health news from the health portion of the Discovery Network.

HealthAnswers.com

http://healthanswers.com/News/News.asp

This site has up to date health news headlines and interesting news stories. Great site!

HealthCentral.com

http://www.healthcentral.com/news/news.cfm

This great website has health news stories related to business, government, wellness, family, sexuality, and alternative medicine among others.

HealthLaw: News

http://www.ljextra.com/practice/health/index.html

HealthLaw has up-to-date news on national health issues from a legal point of view.

HealthWatch

http://www.trufax.org/menu/health1.html

Public health news updates from all over the world.

Intellihealth Online

http://www.intelihealth.com/IH/ihtIH/WSIHW000/333/333.html

Top health news stories from one of the leading online health information companies in the world.

LentilHealth

http://www.lentilhealth.com/

LentilHealth is one place on the internet where you'll find health news from over 2000 online publications, updating as often as every 15 minutes. If it's health and it's happening now, you'll find it on LentilHealth.com.

Mayo Clinic News

http://www.mayohealth.org/home

Health news from the trusted source—the Mayo Clinic.

MSNBC Health News

http://www.msnbc.com/news/HEALTH_Front.asp?a

MSNBC sponsors this great site for recent health news stories.

Nando Times Health and Science News

http://www.nandotimes.com/noframes/healthscience/

This site contains current health news and interesting news from the world of science. Many unique and fascinating stories can be found here each day.

National Clearinghouse for Alcohol and Drug Information News

http://www.health.org/newsroom/

News and press releases on Alcohol and Drug Information.

NewsRX Network

http://www.newsrx.net/dailynews.cgi

This is an incredible database of news stories on all aspects of health and disease.

NPR Health News Stories

http://www.npr.org/news/healthsci/

NPR online health news stories.

Reuters Health Information Services

http://www.reutershealth.com/

Find daily news stories on health and disease. This excellent "first stop" for daily health news is divided into news topics for the health professional and health consumer.

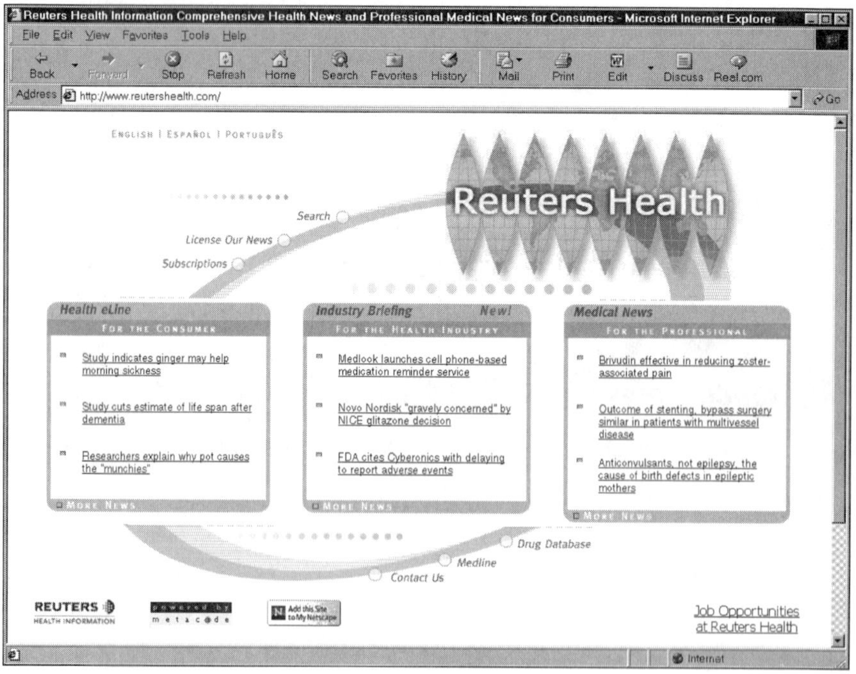

Science Daily

http://www.sciencedaily.com/index.htm

Today's headlines from the latest research news on science and health.

USA Today Health

http://www.medicinenet.com/Script/Main/
HP.asp?li=USA&d=110&cu=16583&w=0

Find health news stories from USA Today.

WebMD Health News Headlines

http://webmd.lycos.com/headlines/

The very popular WebMD's health news source. Excellent resource!

Wellness Newsletter

http://www.wellmedia.com/news.html

A weekly newsletter designed to give you information to improve you mind, body and spirit.

Yahoo! Health News Daily

`http://www.yahoo.com/headlines/health/`

Yahoo!'s news section on daily health stories is another excellent "first stop" for daily health news.

Your Health Daily

`http://199.97.97.16/contWriter/yhd7/`

At this site, find daily health related news stories from the New York Times.

Health Related Searches

100hot.com

`http://www.100hot.com/directory/sports/health.html`

This site ranks the most visited health sites on the entire internet.

About.com Health and Fitness

`http://home.about.com/health/`
`index.htm?IN2PID=938983637.500418&IN2ID=938983637.500418`

This search page will find specific topics for you and has a list of health topics from which to find great health information.

AltaVista Health Topics Search

`http://altavista.looksmart.com/eus1/eus53940/r?l&izf&`

AltaVista is an excellent search engine. Just type the word(s) you want to search in the box.

Ask Jeeves Health Search

http://www.aj.com/main/askjeeves.asp?ask=health&origin=&site_name=Jeeves&metasearch=yes

Ask a question about any aspect of health in the text box and see what comes back for you.

DMOZ—Open Project–Health

http://www.dmoz.org/Health/

This section focuses on topics related to human health and medicine. This is an outstanding resource for great health information.

Dogpile Health Web Catalogue Search

http://catalog.dogpile.com/texis/catalog?c=Health

Web catalogue search results for health.

Environmental Organization Web Directory Search—"Health"

http://www.webdirectory.com/Health/

This is a good search engine that browses the Web for sites that are related to environmental health.

Excite Search—Health and Medicine

http://my.excite.com/lifestyle/health_and_fitness/

Click on one of the health subtopics or use the text box to type in the word(s) for which you would like to search.

Galaxy Search—Health

http://www.einet.net/galaxy/Community/Health.html

At this search engine, click on one of the health subtopics or search through the other health resources such as health articles, events, periodicals, discussion groups, directories, and organizations.

Go2Net Health Search

http://www.go2net.com/channels/health/

Metacrawler health search as well as topical searches by specific health categories.

Go Network Health

http://www.go.com/Center/Health?svx=CTOC_Health

Use this site and its several searches to find excellent health information.

Google Health Search

http://www.google.com/search?q=health

This is a very quick search engine linked to search for health websites.

Health A to Z

http://www.healthatoz.com/

This is an excellent health search—by category or by word search. It includes a large list of health topics which link to many related Web sites.

Infoseek Guide Search—Health

http://guide-p.infoseek.com/Health?tid=1207

This link is designed to be a Web search for all results under the general topic of health. You may make adjustments for additional searching once you have looked at the results. You may also choose from one of the health subtopics listed.

Looksmart—Health

http://www.looksmart.com/eus1/eus317837/eus317920/r?comefrom=nspanel-eus317920

Medical resources for patients and professionals on conditions, health issues, fitness, and community health.

Lycos Search—Health and Medicine

http://dir.lycos.com/Health/

Click on one of the health sub-topics or type in the word(s) for which you would like to search.

Magellan Search—Health and Medicine

`http://magellan.excite.com/health`

Click on one of the health subtopics or type in the word(s) for which you would like to search.

Metahoo—Health Search Robot

`http://metahoo.com/cgi-bin/apexec.pl?etype=odp&template=smart.htm&passurl=/Health/`

Search the web with by choosing one of the health categories or type your topic in the text box.

MedExplorer

`http://www.medexplorer.com/`

This is another great Health and Medical Information Center with a great search engine.

Netscape Health Search

`http://directory.netscape.com/Health/?cp=srpmatcat`

Search the web or ask a question in the text box or choose from among the many health content areas.

Northern Light Search—Health

`http://www.northernlight.com/nlquery.fcg?cb=0&qr=health&orl=`

Type a health topic in the text box or narrow your search with the custom search folders.

Snap—Health Search

`http://www.snap.com/directory/category/0%2C16%2C-7%2C00.html?st.sn.fd.0.dir-7`

NBC and Snap work together to give you a very nifty search engine to help you find health information by categories.

Starting Point Meta Search—Health

`http://www.stpt.com/channel.asp?id=4`

Search for sites that are a bit more holistic health oriented using this search engine.

Virtual Hospital

`http://vh.radiology.uiowa.edu/Misc/Search.html`

With this search engine, simply type the keyword(s) in the box. This engine is designed to be more medically oriented.

WebCrawler Health Topics Search

`http://webcrawler.com/Health/`

Choose from one of the displayed topics or click search and type in the health topic that you seek.

Yahoo Search—Health

`http://www.yahoo.com/Health/`

This site allows you to use the popular Yahoo! search engine to seek health information. Choose one of the health categories listed or type a subject in the box and then click the search button next to the text box.

Health Related Journals, Magazines, and Periodicals

Aesclepian Chronicles

`http://www.forthrt.com/~chronicl/homepage.html`

The goal of the Aesclepian Chronicles is to publish informative and inspirational articles about the many new complementary and allopathic treatment modalities that are emerging. These modalities may be approached from both a personal and a clinical perspective from the Institute of Synergistic Medicine.

Fitness World

http://www.fitnessworld.com

In addition to current issues of the magazine, this site provides information about exercise books and videos, recent news highlights related to health and fitness, and answers to frequently asked questions about fitness. For fitness professionals, it also provides business information and opportunities to exchange with fellow professionals.

Lifelines Newsletter

http://www.lifelines.com/newsletter/frame.html

LifelinesNewsletter is a publication that encourages better health and a better life.

Medscape

http://www.medscape.com/

For health professionals and interested consumers, this newsletter features thousands of full-text, peer-reviewed articles, medical news, Medline, and interactive quizzes. It is updated daily, and free!

Medscape Multispecialty Journal Room

http://www.medscape.com/Home/Topics/multispecialty/directories/dir-MULT.JournalRoom.html

Free access to Medscape's own collection of over 25,000 full-text clinical articles from over 40 journals and more than 15 medical news periodicals.

Men's Fitness On-Line

http://www.mensfitness.com/

This is the online version of the magazine bearing the same name.

New Age Journal On-Line

http://www.newage.com/

New Age Journal is committed to uncovering traditional wisdom and integrating it with modern technology. *New Age Journal* provides more than merely simple information. It is a magazine of insight and perspective, covering people and issues often ignored by the mainstream, and uncovering trends not yet discovered by the more popular press.

New Frontier: Magazine of Transformation

`http://www.newfrontier.com/`

This monthly online newsletter is dedicated to promoting high levels of health and wellness.

New England Journal of Medicine On-Line

`http://www.nejm.org/`

This weekly journal reports the results of important medical research worldwide.

Nutrition Action Healthletter

`http://www.cspinet.org/nah/`

The Center for Science in the Public Interest publishes this health letter.

The Physician and Sports Medicine Online

`http://www.physsportsmed.com/`

This Web site features abstracts from the current issue of the magazine, actual articles from previous issues, a search feature to find selected topics from back issues, and a personal health section with patient-oriented articles on exercise, nutrition, and injury prevention.

The Share Guide Holistic Health Journal and Directory

`http://www.shareguide.com/mag/`

This magazine focuses on holistic health, personal growth, and environmental awareness.

Yoga Journal

`http://www.yogajournal.com/`

This journal is dedicated to communicating the qualities of yoga—peace, integrity, clarity, and compassion—to a broad audience.

Health Research and Evaluation

Carl Uncover

http://www.carl.org/Access.html

Search the largest set of licensed databases in the industry, from local and national newspapers to outstanding sources in business, sciences, technology, medicine, social sciences, the arts, consumer information, patents, education and reference sources, along with the online public access catalog and any Z39.50 library catalog on the Web.

Combined Health Information Database

http://chid.nih.gov/

CHID is a database produced by health-related agencies of the Federal Government. It provides titles, abstracts, and availability information for health information and health education resources. The value of this database is that it lists a wealth of health promotion and education - materials and program descriptions that are not indexed elsewhere. New records are added quarterly and current listings are checked regularly to help ensure that all entries are up to date and still available from their original sources. Some older records are retained for archival purposes.

Electronic Resources for Evaluators

http://it.usu.edu/itrs/AEA/index.html

Incredible resource page for health research and evaluation.

ERIC Clearinghouse on Assessment and Evaluation

http://ericae.net/

ERIC looks for journal articles that are a bit more related but not limited to education.

FindArticles.com

http://www.findarticles.com/PI/index.jhtml

Search for quality articles in more than 300 reputable magazines and journals.

Healthfinder On-line Publications

http://www.healthfinder.gov/moretools/

Many of the best federal consumer health information publications available online are included in the healthfinder database. Search for online publications, publications catalogs, and Web sites featuring electronic documents.

Healthgate

http://www.healthgate.com/

The objective of Healthgate is to make information access and coverage both thorough and easy, while maintaining the highest standards of academic and scientific integrity.

Medline

http://www.healthgate.com/HealthGate/MEDLINE/search.shtml

Search through Medline for peer-reviewed journal articles on most aspects of health and disease.

NYU Health Education Professional Resources

http://www.nyu.edu/education/hepr/resources/online/index.html

This page contains another excellent list of links to health related research resources online.

Steve Gabeny's (Indiana State) huge list of Community Health Bookmarks

http://web.indstate.edu/hlthsfty/ch/bkmrks.htm

Look under the Research and Planning Section.

Alternative Medicine and Holistic Health

part
2

Acupuncture.com

http://www.Acupuncture.com/

At this site, find traditional oriental therapies along with related resources for consumers, practitioners, and students. The site also includes other related information and links as well.

Alternative Medicine Foundation

http://www.amfoundation.org/

This site provides responsible and reliable information for patients and consumers as well as evidence-based research resources for health care professionals.

Alternative Medicine Home Page

http://www.pitt.edu/~cbw/altm.html

This site is a jumpstation for sources of information on unconventional, unorthodox, unproven, or alternative, complementary, innovative, and integrative therapies.

Alternative Medicine Links

http://www.altmedicine.com/

This site links to some of the most helpful alternative, complementary, and preventive health news pages on the Internet.

Alternative Medicine Weekly

http://www.americanwholehealth.com/

Studies conducted using alternative medicine are listed weekly from this excellent Web site. Drop in regularly.

American Holistic Health Association

http://ahha.org/

The American Holistic Health Association (AHHA) is the leading national resource connecting people with vital soulutions for reaching a higher level of wellness.

American Massage Therapy Association

http://www.amtamassage.org/

The mission of the American Massage Therapy Association is to develop and advance the art, science, and practice of massage therapy in a caring, professional, and ethical manner in order to promote the health and welfare of humanity. Visit the site of this most popular form of complementary health care.

Dream Up, Dream Links

http://www.dreamup.com/

This site contains nearly everything you could want to know about the magical world of dreaming.

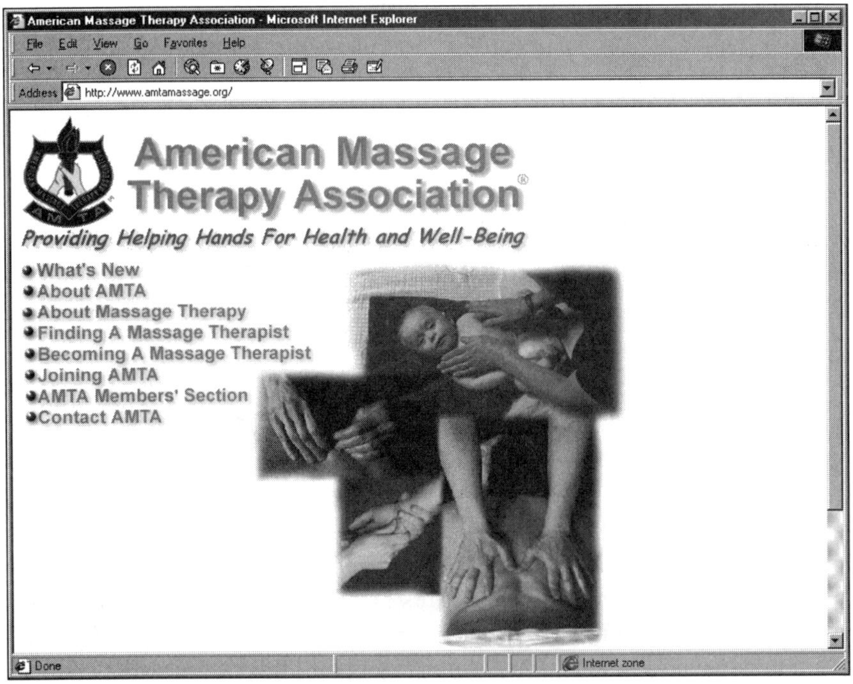

part 2

Herbal Information Center

http://www.kcweb.com/herb/herbmain.htm

Here, you will find descriptions of the most common herbs, and how they can be used to treat today's health problems.

HerbNET

http://www.herbnet.com/

This site claims to be the most comprehensive site on the Web for those seeking information on herbs, herb products and remedies, herb publications...in fact, everything herbal can be found here!

Herb Research (Foundation) News

http://www.herbs.org/index.html

This site contains research and education on worldwide use of herbs for health, environmental conservation, and international development.

Holistic Healing Web Page

http://www.holisticmed.com/

This Web page has extensive holistic health related information, including articles, Web links, group links, and mailing information lists.

Homeopathy Home Page

http://www.homeopathyhome.com/

This page is a jumping off point and aims to provide links to every resource available related to homeopathy. There are FAQs, a reference library, discussion groups, and more.

The International Advocates for Health Freedom

http://www.iahf.com/

The creators of this page describe themselves as a catalytic entity designed to foster networking between health freedom activists worldwide in order to foster opposition to the elements of coercion: the UN's International Council of Drug Regulating Authorities, and all regulating bodies falling under its auspices including the FDA, TGA, HPB, MCA, MCC, and others.

Near-death Experience Research Foundation

http://www.nderf.org/

Great page on the strange phenomenon of the NDE.

Office of Alternative Medicine at the National Institutes of Health

http://nccam.nih.gov/

Office of Alternative Medicine (OAM) identifies and evaluates unconventional health care practices. The OAM supports and conducts research and research training on these practices and disseminates information.

Oxygen and Ozone Therapies

http://www.oxytherapy.com/

Find information on oxygen therapies including, the use of hydrogen peroxide, ozone therapy, hyperbaric oxygen, stabilized oxygen, and ionization.

Spirit WWW

http://www.spiritweb.org/

This site lists spirituality resources on the WWW, including links to many forms of spirituality.

Wellspring Media

http://wellmedia.com/links.html

Excellent website relating to holistic thinking, spirituality, and personal development.

Cancer

American Cancer Society

http://www.cancer.org/

The official home page for the ACS provides information concerning the symptoms, treatment, and prevention of cancer.

American Institute for Cancer Research

http://www.aicr.org/

The nation's leading charity in the field of diet, nutrition and cancer prevention.

Cancer Care Inc.

http://www.cancercareinc.org/

This cancer-related Web site lists Internet- and telephone-based support services, as well as information on counseling, local physician referrals, and even financial assistance. Online forums allow patients to converse with experts.

Cancer News on the Net

http://www.cancernews.com/

This site is dedicated to bringing patients and their families the latest information on cancer diagnosis and treatment.

Cancer Prevention Research Center

http://www.uri.edu/research/cprc/

The primary mission of the Cancer Research Center is to enhance the quality and quantity of life through prevention of cancer, other chronic diseases and premature death. The primary means is through basic and applied research and dissemination of our most effective behavior change technologies.

CanSearch

http://www.cansearch.org/canserch/canserch.htm

The purpose of this guide is to assist those not experienced in finding sources on the Net to go to cancer resources quickly and find answers to their questions or at least become more informed patients and caretakers.

InterNet Resources for Cancer

http://www.ncl.ac.uk/~nchwww/guides/clinks1.htm

This guide contains over 30 pages of links to cancer-related information. Many sites contain information for both the public and health professionals.

JOMOL Cancer Research Information

`http://www.jomol.regensburg.com/`

This site provides information on an alternative therapy for cancer.

National Cancer Institute

`http://cancernet.nci.nih.gov/pdqfull.html`

This is the complete information source of the National Cancer Institute. The National Cancer Institute (NCI) is a component of the National Institutes of Health (NIH), one of eight agencies that compose the Public Health Service (PHS) in the Department of Health and Human Services (DHHS). The NCI, established under the National Cancer Act of 1937, is the Federal Government's principal agency for cancer research and training.

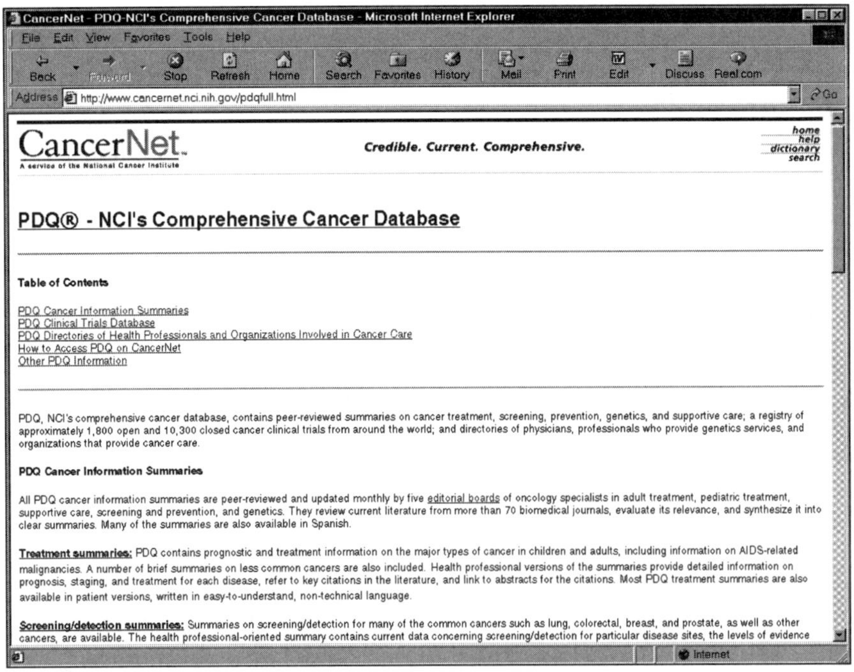

National Comprehensive Cancer Network

http://www.cancer.med.umich.edu/NCCN/NCCN.html

The NCCN was formed to create cancer-management strategies for large employers and third-party payers. Its mission is to integrate the experience of member cancer centers to ensure delivery of high quality, cost-effective services to cancer patients across the country.

Skin Cancer Information Page

http://www.maui.net/~southsky/introto.html

This thorough information page on skin cancer is designed to be a gathering place for all available information about skin cancer and related subjects.

Steve Dunn's Cancer Information Page

http://cancerguide.org/

This informative guide is dedicated to helping the user find the answers to questions about cancer, and especially to helping find what questions to ask.

University of Pennsylvania Cancer Resource

http://www.oncolink.upenn.edu/

This extensive Web site is touted as the first multimedia oncology information resource on the Internet.

Yahoo!'s Cancer Links

http://www.yahoo.com/Health/Diseases_and_Conditions/Cancer/

A thorough search of the Internet's Web sites devoted to information on the various types of cancer can be found here.

Community Health Education

American Heart Association National Center

http://www.americanheart.org/

The American Heart Association is one of the world's premier health organizations, and is committed to reducing disability and death from cardiovascular diseases and stroke. This site provides a wealth of information almost 300 subjects from the American Heart Association.

Center for Disease Control and Prevention

http://www.cdc.gov/cdc.html

The CDC's mission is to promote health and quality of life by preventing and controlling disease, injury, and disability. This site contains links to other agencies, and a lot of information on various health related topics such as, the CDC, health information, travelers' health, publications and products, data and statistics, training and employment, and funding.

Community Health Concepts Home Page

http://web.indstate.edu/hlthsfty/ch/ch.htm

This page includes community health courses with outlines, excellent information and a huge list of community health related links. This is a great resource.

Community Toolbox

http://ctb.lsi.ukans.edu/

Outstanding resource for all aspects of community health and development.

Escoffery's Health Education Page

http://userwww.service.emory.edu/~cescoff/cam.html

A jumpsite to resources on Certified Health Education Specialist (C.H.E.S.), professional organizations, health education/public health conference calendar, health information resources, health education and promotion listservs, public health software, schools of public health, health resources, and state health addresses on the Internet.

National Center for Health Statistics

http://www.cdc.gov/nchs/about.htm

NCHS is the Federal Government's principal vital and health statistics agency.

National Health Information Center

http://nhic-nt.health.org/

NHIC is a health information referral service which puts health professionals and consumers who have health questions in touch with those organizations that are best able to provide answers. This is a great resource for health publications, announcements, and access to 1,100 health organizations and government offices.

National Institutes of Health

http://www.nih.gov/

Great information about the NIH, health information, news and events, grants and contracts, scientific research and more.

NewsFile

http://www.homepage.holowww.com/

This site contains references and abstracts to news and journal articles that relate to public and community health. Excellent resource for research.

Pan American Health Organization

http://www.paho.org/

PAHO's mission is to cooperate technically with the Member Countries and to stimulate cooperation among them in order that, while maintaining a healthy environment and charting a course to sustainable human development, the peoples of the Americas may achieve Health for All and by All.

World Health Association

http://www.who.ch/

The objective of WHO is the attainment by all peoples of the highest possible level of health. Health, as defined in the WHO Constitution, is a state of complete physical, mental and social well-being and not merely the absence of disease or infirmity.

Diseases: Chronic and Acute

American Diabetes Association

http://www.diabetes.org/

This is the homepage of the American Diabetes Association. Their mission is to prevent and cure diabetes and to improve the lives of all people affected by diabetes.

American Lung Association

http://www.lungusa.org/

This is the ALA online resource for information on asthma and other lung diseases, tobacco control, and environmental health.

CDC Diseases Page

http://www.cdc.gov/

Information on many diseases in the United States including data on incidence and prevalence of diseases.

Chronic Illness-Net

http://www.chronicillnet.org/

This website describes itself as the first multimedia information source on the Internet dedicated to chronic illnesses including AIDS, cancer, Persian Gulf War Syndrome, autoimmune diseases, Chronic Fatigue Syndrome, heart disease and neurological diseases.

CliniWeb International

http://www.ohsu.edu/cliniweb/C.html

Database for all diseases. Like an encyclopedia only better.

Diseases, Disorders, and Related Topics

http://www.mic.ki.se/Diseases/index.html

Diseases, Disorders and Related Topics Resources on the Internet for laypersons, health care professionals and scientists. Gigantic Resource—Excellent place to begin searching for disease information.

Med Help General Library

http://medhlp.netusa.net/

This page links to thousands (seemingly) of articles covering a wide variety of diseases, conditions, and health concerns.

Morbidity and Mortality Weekly Report

http://www.cdc.gov/epo/mmwr/mmwr.html

The Morbidity and Mortality Weekly Report (MMWR) Series is prepared by the Centers for Disease Control and Prevention (CDC) and are based on weekly reports to CDC by state health departments.

Mother Nature's General Store: Health Library

http://www.mothernature.com/

A general health information library that includes information on AIDS and cancer.

Patient's Guide to Healthcare Information on the Internet

http://www3.bc.sympatico.ca/me/patientsguide/

Here's a step-by-step guide to locating and researching medical conditions on the Internet.

Rethinking AIDS Website

http://www.virusmyth.com/aids/index.htm

Is the AIDS virus harmless? Is AIDS not contagious? Are the AIDS tests worthless? Is AIDS medication killing patients? Find out what the AIDS establishment and media do not want you to know. Worth looking over.

Virology WWW server

http://www.bocklabs.wisc.edu/Welcome.html

This website is a huge resource collecting all possible information related to viruses including maps of viruses, digitized images of viruses, conferences, news and journals, links, emerging Infectious Diseases and more.

WebMD Health

http://my.webmd.com/condition_center_all

Diseases & Conditions information from this award winning health website.

Yahoo: Diseases and Conditions

http://www.yahoo.com/Health/Diseases_and_Conditions/

Yahoo search for websites on the internet that are disease related.

Environmental Health

Agency for Toxic Substances and Disease Registry

http://atsdr1.atsdr.cdc.gov:8080/cx.html

A simple guide to search the World Wide Web for environmental health information, the Registry's primary focus is to find and share global information resources with the public on the linkage between human exposure to hazardous chemicals and adverse human health effects.

National Center for Environmental Health (NCEH)

http://www.cdc.gov/nceh/ncehhome.htm

The mission of the NCEH is to provide national leadership through science and service, and to promote health and quality of life by preventing and controlling disease, birth defects, disability, and death resulting from interactions between people and their environment.

National Institute of Environmental Health Sciences

http://www.niehs.nih.gov/

The mission of the National Institute of Environmental Health Sciences (NIEHS) is to reduce the burden of human illness and dysfunction from environmental causes by understanding each of these elements and how they interrelate.

Project NatureConnect

http://www.pacificrim.net/~nature/

This page is especially for nature enthusiasts. The designers of this page created this site to help others promote a heightened sense of self-worth and environmental responsibility.

Yahoo! Search on Environmental Health

http://www.yahoo.com/Health/Environmental_Health/

Search multiple sites, links, and home pages as well as information on environmental health.

Exercise and Fitness

American Alliance for Health, Physical Education, Recreation, and Dance

http://www.aahperd.org/

AAHPERD's home page includes links to American Association for Active Lifestyles and Fitness, American Association for Health Education, American Association for Leisure and Recreation, National Association for Girls and Women in Sport, National Association for Sport and Physical Education, and the National Dance Association.

American College of Sports Medicine

http://www.acsm.org/

This is the home page of the largest, most respected sports medicine and exercise science organization in the world.

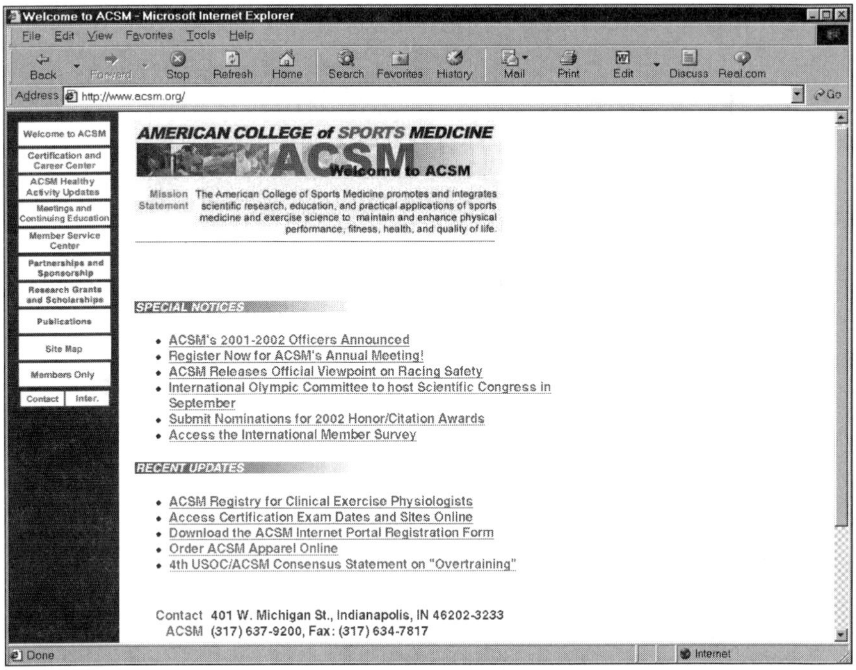

American Council on Exercise

`http://www.acefitness.org/`

This nonprofit organization sets certification standards for exercise professionals and runs a consumer fitness hotline offering referrals to ACE certified personal trainers. The Web site features information about its programs, referrals to fitness resources, and news about exercise and fitness.

Bicycling Information

`http://www.cascade.org/links.html`

This site is loaded with bicycling Web sites all over the world. Nearly anything a user might want to know regarding bicycling can be accessed from this page.

Dr. Pribut's Running Injuries Page

`http://www.clark.net/pub/pribut/spsport.html`

This site contains information about running and about preventing and treating many types of running injuries.

Exercise, Fitness and Pregnancy

http://www.noah.cuny.edu/pregnancy/march_of_dimes/pre_preg.plan/fit42is.html

A lot of information on exercise and pregnancy, including benefits, risks, and guidelines can be found at this site.

Fitness Products Council

http://www.sportlink.com/fitness/

This site contains a Speakers Bureau, market research reports, a news letter, and the Surgeon General's recent report on health, fitness, and exercise.

National Coalition for Promoting Physical Activity

http://www.ncppa.org/

This premier organization promotes physical activity. The objective of NCPPA is to unite the strengths of public, private and industry efforts into a collaborative partnership to inspire Americans to lead physically active lifestyles to enhance their health and quality of life.

New Zealand Fitness Home Page

http://home.ait.ac.nz/staff/pmellow//

This outstanding resource includes links and information on fitness, sports, and health through exercise.

The Physician and Sports Medicine Online

http://www.physsportsmed.com/

This Web site features abstracts from the current issue of the magazine, actual articles from previous issues, a search feature to find selected topics from back issues, and a Personal Health section with patient-oriented articles on exercise, nutrition, and injury prevention.

Road Runners Club of America

http://www.rrca.org/

Novice and experienced runners alike will find a vast array of information provided by this not-for-profit organization, including a calendar of events, guidelines for putting on a race, how to start a club, and tips for running safely.

The Running Page

http://sunsite.unc.edu/drears/running/running.html

The Running Page contains information about upcoming races, race results, places to run, running related products, magazines, and other information.

Runner's World Online

http://www.runnersworld.com/

This site contains a wide variety of information about running, including tips for beginning runners, advice about training, and a shoe buyer's guide.

WWW Women's Sports Page

http://fiat.gslis.utexas.edu/~lewisa/womsprt.html

The Women's Sports Page is an excellent jumpsite to women's sports pages around the WWW. Some of the topics include women's sports, women's sports organizations, and issues in women's sports.

General Health

America Online (AOL) Health Center

http://www.aol.com/webcenters/health/home.adp

Site includes all types of health information including news, health assessments, and lots of reference information. Great site!

Clearinghouse—Health and Medicine

http://www.clearinghouse.net/cgi-bin/chadmin/viewcat/Health___Medicine?kywd++

This page is an enormous resource of a very wide range of health topics. Choose one and then click the hypertext link to up-to-date information.

Duke University Healthy Devil: On-line

http://h-devil-www.mc.duke.edu/h-devil

This general health resource location from Duke University contains a large list of health topics with basic definitions.

Alice

http://www.cc.columbia.edu/cu/healthwise/

The Go Ask Alice page has interactive answers to questions on various health topics.

Hardin Meta Directory for Internet Health Information

http://www.arcade.uiowa.edu/hardin-www/md.html

This directory points to the most complete and frequently cited lists in many health subjects—a bit more medically oriented, but good.

HealthAnswers.Com

http://healthanswers.com/

A very good guide to health information.

Healthtouch

http://www.healthtouch.com/

Healthtouch offers information on dozens of health topics and diseases as well as a medication guide on drug uses, precautions, and side effects.

Health World Online

http://www.healthy.net/

Provides 10 categories of health and wellness topics for consumers and professionals including nutrition, mind-body connection, and a medical library.

Johns Hopkins Health Information

http://www.intelihealth.com/IH/ihtIH?t=408&st=408&r=WSIHW000

Intellihealth Home. Great starting point for nearly any health information.

KidsHealth

http://www.kidshealth.org/index2.html

A mighty Web site devoted to the health of children and teens created by the medical experts at the Nemours Foundation, KidsHealth has trainloads of accurate, up-to-date information about growth, food, fitness, childhood infections, immunizations, lab tests, medical and surgical conditions, and the latest treatments. You'll find health games, How the Body Works animations, the KidsVote health poll, and tons of surprises. So get on board and explore!

The Longevity Game

http://www.northwesternmutual.com/games/longevity/

See how old you'll be before you pass on.

Mediconsult.com, Inc.

http://www.mediconsult.com/

This health website is one of the most complete and comprehensive health and medical info pages on the net. It gathers up-to-date information on all topics of health from journal reviews to the latest news. This is a great website. Spend some time here and you will be amazed.

National Council Against Health Fraud, Inc. (NCAHF)

http://www.ncahf.org/

The health information watchdog NCAHF is a nonprofit, tax-exempt, voluntary health agency that focuses its attention on health fraud, mis information, and quackery as public health problems.

Patient's Guide to Healthcare Information on the Internet

http://www3.bc.sympatico.ca/me/patientsguide/

Here's a step-by-step guide to locating and researching medical conditions on the Internet.

You First

http://www.youfirst.com/

This is a highly personalized, confidential, and interactive opportunity to determine your health risks with free online health risk appraisal. The Web site includes links to seasonal health tips, America's health risks, top 10 causes of death, and answers to frequently asked questions.

Governmental Health Resources

Administration for Children and Families

http://www.acf.dhhs.gov/

ACF is responsible for federal programs that promote the economic and social well-being of families, children, individuals, and communities

Department of Health and Human Services

http://www.hhs.gov/

DHHS is the United States government's principal agency for protecting the health of all Americans and providing essential human services, especially for those who are least able to help themselves

Food and Drug Administration (FDA)

http://www.fda.gov/

FDA's mission is to promote and protect the public health by helping safe and effective products reach the market in a timely way, and monitoring products for continued safety after they are in use.

Health Care Financing Administration

http://www.hcfa.gov/

HCFA provides health insurance for over 74 million Americans through Medicare, Medicaid and SCHIP.

Health Resources and Services Administration

`http://www.hrsa.dhhs.gov/`

Publications, resources and referrals on health care services for low-income, uninsured individuals and those with special health care needs.

Healthy People 2010

`http://www.health.gov/healthypeople/`

This page contains the official government document regarding U.S. health goals and objectives for the year 2010; includes special population health risks for older adults, women, and minorities.

US National Library of Medicine

`http://www.nlm.nih.gov/`

The largest medical library and creator of Medline

Health and Disease Care

AMSO Managed Care Forum

`http://www.amso.com/`

The purpose of the AMSO Web page is to provide a forum for healthcare professionals and consumers of healthcare to learn and expound about the everchanging managed healthcare industry.

CenterWatch Clinical Trials Listing Service

`http://www.centerwatch.com/`

You can use this listing to search for clinical trials, find out information about physicians and medical centers performing clinical research, and to learn about drug therapies newly approved by the Food and Drug Administration.

Convergent Medical Systems

http://www.convergentmedical.com/

This site has information relating to healthcare consultants, strategic, managed care, health policy planning, health insurance, medical education, medical regulation, health promotion, wellness programs, allied health professions, alternative and complementary medicine, and world medicine.

GlobalMedic

http://www.globalmedic.com/

Empowering healthcare users through education and prevention, this interesting site includes a medical encyclopedia, nutrition information, and health information for women and children.

LIFE: Life and Health Insurance Information Site

http://www.life-line.org/

An excellent educational site designed to provide you with straightforward, unbiased information on life and health insurance.

Medscape

http://www.medscape.com/Home/About.html

Medscape pools information from clinical journals, medical news providers, medical education programs, and material created expressly for Medscape. The result is a medical Web site rich in content, broad in appeal, and high in quality.

Yahoo! Internet Search—Health Care

http://www.yahoo.com/Health/Health_Care/

This is a full Internet search of all things related to health care using the Yahoo! search engine.

Health Education (School)

ERIC Clearinghouse on Teaching and Teacher Education

http://www.ericsp.org/

A great site for information and internet resources for education, teachers, teachers organizations, publications, financial aid, professional development schools, educational materials and resources and more.

ERIC Clearinghouse on Teaching and Teacher Education: Health, Physical Education, Recreation and Dance Divisions

http://www.ericsp.org/pages/healthpe/index.html

ERIC's homepage (see previous listing) in specialty areas listed in title.

ETA Update

http://eta.aed.org/

Tips for implementing CDC School Health Education guidelines.

The Health Education Hitlist

http://www.ex.ac.uk/~dregis/healthy.html

A jumpsite to World Wide Web pages for those interested in health education including, indices and search engines, school health resource services, health education, health care, public health, and other health issues.

PE Central Health Lesson Ideas and Plans

http://www.pecentral.org/lessonideas/health/healthlp.html

Excellent resource for anyone who teaches health and wellness classes. Site contains lesson plans and ideas to supplement a class.

Health Organizations

AAHPERD

http://www.aahperd.org/

The American Alliance for Health, Physical Education, Recreation & Dance (AAHPERD) has promoted quality education programs to improve Americans' total health and fitness.

American Association for Retired Persons

http://www.aarp.org/

AARP is a reputable nonprofit organization dedicated to securing the rights of older adults. A wide variety of links serve the health advocacy and informational needs of older adults.

American College Health Association

http://www.acha.org/

The American College Health Association is a national nonprofit organization serving and representing the interests of professionals and students in health and higher education.

American School Health Association

http://www.ashaweb.org/

Promoting the health of our nation's youth

Association for Worksite Health Promotion

http://www.awhp.org/

This is a professional organization for worksite health promoters. The home page offers directions for becoming a member and information about conferences.

Health Promotion

Association for Worksite Health Promotion

http://www.awhp.org/

AWHP is a not-for-profit network of worksite health promotion professionals dedicated to sharing the best-of-practice methods, processes and technologies. Site includes information on AWHP as well as other resources and links to wellness, health and fitness pages.

Institute of Health Promotion Research

http://www.ihpr.ubc.ca/

Its mission is to provide a UBC focus for interdisciplinary collaboration on research, education, and community partnerships in health promotion.

Monash Health Promotion on the Internet

http://www.monash.edu.au/health/

Australia's Monash University's page on health promotion features a health promotion interactive lounge, and information and sites for the following: patient education, calendar of health events, Internet health directory, health resources, and health promotion research and education.

Office of Disease Prevention and Health Promotion

http://odphp.osophs.dhhs.gov/

ODPHP works to strengthen the disease prevention and health promotion priorities within the collaborative framework of the HHS agencies

Rural Health Resources

http://www.siu.edu/~crhssd/rhres.htm

The SIU center for Rural Health and Social Service Development is an excellent site with information and links to many great resources, including rural health resources, health agencies, medical resources, publications, socioeconomic data resources, search engines, and Web page and HTML help guides.

Wellness Councils of America (WELCOA)

http://www.welcoa.org/

The Wellness Councils of America (WELCOA) is a national nonprofit membership organization dedicated to promoting healthier lifestyles, especially through health promotion activities at the worksite.

Health Psychology

Alcoholics Anonymous Resources: A Collection of AA Information

http://www.recovery.org/aa/

Find information and links on many aspects of AA, including literature, history, intergroup phone numbers, meetings, conventions, computer programs, and links to more AA related resources.

American Psychological Association

http://www.apa.org/

This is the home page of the APA. It includes the newspaper of the American Psychological Association, as well as other links and information to books, journals, employment, public practice, education information, and much more.

As a Man Thinketh

http://www.concentric.net/~conure/allen.html

The entire text of this fantastic little book is online.

At Health Inc.

http://www.athealth.com/

At Health Inc. is a site designed to connect mental health professionals and those they serve with the power and the resources of the Internet.

Centre for Psychotherapeutic Studies

http://www.shef.ac.uk/~psysc/psychotherapy/index.html

Search all of the major mental health resources on the World Wide Web from one page; connect to all 857 psychology, psychiatry, neuroscience, and social science journals and journal search engines; locate mental health texts, search for a colleague, a quotation, an electronic book, define a word, find a synonym, consult an electronic biography, or connect to all of the major Internet search engines. This site is remarkable!

Consciousness/Parapsychology/Transpersonal Psychology

http://www.uwsp.edu/acad/psych/dk/danielpg.htm

This is a very interesting page by a professor at University of Wisconsin–Stevens Point. His emphases and the links on this page are devoted to consciousness, altered states of consciousness, parapsychology, and transpersonal psychology.

Infinity Institute International

http://www.infinityinst.com/

Infinity Institute International is an excellent resource on hypnosis and self-hypnosis.

Magic Stream

http://fly.hiwaay.net/~garson/

This site includes the *Journal of Emotional Wellness*. The Web Dex contains extensive links on topics such as addictions, recovery, child abuse, fitness, nutrition, depression, family, and more. The *Journal* contains original poetry, essays, articles, and short stories focused on personal growth and the universal in human emotion.

Mental Health.com

http://www.mentalhealth.com/main.html

Internet Mental Health is a free encyclopedia of mental health information along with loads of other resources regarding mental health.

Mental Health Net

http://www.cmhc.com/

A comprehensive guide to mental health online, featuring over 7,000 resources, this site has information on disorders such as depression, anxiety, panic attacks, chronic fatigue syndrome, substance abuse, professional resources in psychology, psychiatry and social work, journals, and self-help magazines.

Mental Health Search

http://mentalhealth.about.com/health/mentalhealth/library/blsearch.htm

About.Com's excellent resource for finding all things related to stress management and mental & emotional health.

Sleep Medicine Home Page

http://www.cloud9.net/~thorpy/

This home page lists resources regarding all aspects of sleep, including, the physiology of sleep, clinical sleep medicine, sleep research, federal and state information, patient information, and business-related groups.

Spiritual Consciousness

http://www.nerdworld.com/users/dstein/nw142.html

This is an enormous resource of spiritual health related Web sites around the world.

The Taoism Information Page

http://www.clas.ufl.edu/users/gthursby/taoism/

This page contains almost everything relevant to the philosophy of Taoism.

Zen Stories to Tell Your Neighbors

http://www.rider.edu/users/suler/zenstory/zenstory.html

This is a very nice collection of thought provoking Zen stories. Zensational!

Heart Health

American Heart Association

http://www.americanheart.org/

This site provides information on hundreds of topics relating to cardiovascular health and disease, including cardiorespiratory endurance exercise.

Can Heart Disease Really Be Prevented?

http://www.cardio.com/articles/preventn.htm

By Peter M. Abel, M.D., medical director of the Prevention Center for Cardiovascular Disease at the Cardiovascular Institute of the South/ Morgan City, this site has excellent information and links to many other resources on heart disease.

Cardiovascular Institute of the South

http://www.cardio.com/

CIS, a leading center for the advanced diagnosis and treatment of heart and circulatory disease, presents a wide-ranging library of doctor column-style reports on this vital and rapidly evolving aspect of medicine. These reports cover the full spectrum of prevention, diagnosis, and nonsurgical and surgical treatment of circulatory problems.

Franklin Science Institute

http://www.fi.edu/biosci/heart.html

This site provides learning opportunities about how the heart functions in an interactive lab simulation. This is a very interesting website on the heart.

Healthy Heart

http://sln.fi.edu/biosci/healthy/healthy.html

Excellent information on a wide range subjects pertaining to a healthy heart including educational and enrichment activities.

Late Breaking News for Heart Health

`http://www.mindspring.com/~mtm/news.html`

This site is dedicated to natural health, alternative medicine, and the latest available news related to the improvement of overall health of men and women over 35.

The Learning Center

`http://www.hsforum.com/frameset1.asp?loc=learningctr.asp`

Heart Disease and your health—what you should know. This page provides information and explanations of common cardiovascular diseases specifically for the non-medical audience.

Linus C. Pauling

`http://www.internetwks.com/pauling/`

This interesting Web page lists extensive information on reversing heart disease without surgery. It follows much of the theories and ideas espoused by the late Linus Pauling.

Vegetarian Diets

`http://www.fatfree.com/FAQ/ada-paper`

This page contains a position paper by the American Dietetic Association. It states the Association's summary of the healthful nature of a vegetarian diet.

Nutrition

American Dietetics Association Home Page

`http://www.eatright.org/`

A site designed to promote optimal nutrition, health, and well-being, this Web page contains nutrition information and resources.

The American Heart Association Diet

http://www.americanheart.org/catalog/Health_catpage4.html

This eating plan from the American Heart Association describes the latest advice of medical and nutritional experts. The best way to help lower your blood cholesterol is to eat less saturated fatty acids and cholesterol and control your weight. The AHA Diet gives you an easy-to-follow guide to eating with your heart in mind.

Arbor Communications Nutrition Resources on the Internet

http://arborcom.com/

This site contains one of the most comprehensive lists available of Internet nutrition resources.

Ask the Dietitian

http://www.dietitian.com/

This is a question-and-answer page on nearly all aspects of nutrition.

Aspartame (Nutrasweet) Toxicity Information Center

http://www.holisticmed.com/aspartame/

With detailed scientific and general documentation regarding the toxicity of Nutrasweet, Equal, Diet Coke, Diet Pepsi, and other aspartame-containing items, this Web page includes real life reports of acute and chronic toxicity due to long-term ingestion. Also included is extensive scientific and general information and resources.

Diet and Weight Loss/Fitness Home Page

http://www1.mhv.net/~donn/diet.html

This great site offers FAQs about dieting, weight loss tips from readers, weight tables comparison study, news wire summaries, all about calories, and multiple links to Ask the Dietitian, Artificial Sweetener Controversy, Vegetarians, and many others. There are also links to fitness sites and information on support groups.

Center for Science in the Public interest

http://www.cspinet.org/

A page designed to promote health by educating the public about nutrition and alcohol.

CyberDiet

http://www.cyberdiet.com/

This page is highly interactive providing an individualized dietary planner with a searchable database, dietary assessment tools, and food planners.

Electronic Gourmet Guide

http://www.globalgourmet.com/

This is a very tantalizing page with a lot of interesting information on food.

Fast Food Facts—Interactive Food Finder

http://www.olen.com/food/

This wonderful page is designed to help anyone determine the ingredients of his or her favorite fast foods. Interactive and useful.

Food and Nutrition: Selected Electronic Resources

http://www.nalusda.gov/fnic/

This excellent Web site may be the first place to search for anything related to food and nutrition.

The Food Pyramid

http://www.ganesa.com/food/index.html

Find up-to-date information on the latest information on what we used to know as the four food groups.

Health and Nutrition

http://dinnercoop.cs.cmu.edu/dinnercoop/special/health.html

This page is filled with a large number of more links to nutrition information around the world.

International Food Information Council

`http://ificinfo.health.org/`

This page is designed to enhance consumers' abilities to make informed food choices by developing and supporting informational and educational programs on food safety, nutrition and health. It includes a lot of good information relating to healthy hearts.

My Menus

`http://www.mymenus.com/`

My Menus is the best recipe site on the Web! There are thousands of nutritional recipes and complete nutritional information. Instantly custom-build your own meal plans. Look up recipes by nutritional characteristic. YUMMY STUFF!

Nutrition.gov

`http://www.nutrition.gov/home/index.php3`

A new federal resource, provides easy access to all online federal government information on nutrition. This national resource makes obtaining government information on nutrition, healthy eating, physical activity, and food safety, easily accessible in one place for many Americans.

Nutribase On-Line

`http://www.nutribase.com/`

This site features an interactive online database of over 19,000 food items and their associated nutrient information. A user can view, rank, query, and search by food names. The database includes more than 3,000 menu items from over 70 restaurants. This site also features a weight-loss calculator, a calorie requirements calculator, desirable weight and body fat content charts, a directory of 1,400 food and supplement makers, a listing of healthy food substitutions, a glossary of foods and cooking terms, toll-free numbers for food makers, and 1,000 quotes and tips for dieters. It's all here!

Professional Resources in Nutrition Science

http://academic.brooklyn.cuny.edu/hns/prins/

This page is a service provided by the Brooklyn College Nutrition Faculty and Students! This homepage is designed for nutrition professionals and students to access information useful for professional practice in nutrition. A great resource.

Veggies Unite!

http://www.vegweb.com/

This is a central site for all things vegetarian.

Public Health

APHA

http://www.apha.org/

This is the home page for the American Public Health Association.

Career Espresso!

http://www.sph.emory.edu/studentservice/Career.html

Career Espresso! is the absolute hottest public health career search Web site anywhere

NewsFile

http://www.newsrx.net/home.cgi

This site contains references and abstracts to journal articles that relate to public and community health. Excellent resource for research.

The Virtual Public Health Center

http://www-sci.lib.uci.edu/~martindale/PHealth.html

This Web site is possibly the most comprehensive resource out there on public health.

Safety and Injury Prevention

Amazing Environmental Organization WebDirectory

`http://www.webdirectory.com/`

A huge directory of web sites for all sorts of environmental subjects including those relating to safety.

Bicycle Helmet Safety Institute

`http://www.bhsi.org/index.htm`

This small, active, nonprofit, consumer-funded program acts as a clearinghouse and a technical resource for bicycle helmet information. It includes information on statistics, publications, laws, and advice on bicycle helmet safety as well as other helmet- and bicycle-type links.

Consumer Product Safety Commission

`gopher://cpsc.gov/`

The U.S. Consumer Product Safety Commission (CPSC), is an independent federal regulatory agency that was created in 1972 by Congress in the Consumer Product Safety Act. This gopher server contains lots of information and links regarding consumer product safety.

The Injury Prevention Web

`http://www.injurypreventionweb.org/`

A service of the Center for Childhood Injury Prevention and the State and Territorial Injury Prevention Directors' Association. Excellent resource.

The National Institute of Environmental Health Sciences

`http://www.niehs.nih.gov/`

NIEHS mission is to reduce the burden of human illness and dysfunction from environmental causes by understanding each of these elements and how they interrelate. The NIEHS achieves its mission through multidisciplinary biomedical research programs, prevention and intervention efforts, and communication strategies that encompass training, education, technology transfer, and community outreach.

National Institute for Occupational Safety and Health (NIOSH)

`http://www.cdc.gov/niosh/homepage.html`

NIOSH is part of the Centers for Disease Control and Prevention (CDC) and is responsible for conducting research and making recommendations for the prevention of work-related illness and injuries.

National Safety Council

`http://www.nsc.org/`

National Safety Council's mission is to educate and influence society to adopt safety, health, and environmental policies, practices, and procedures that prevent and mitigate human suffering and economic losses arising from preventable causes.

Product Safety Link Directory

`http://www.safetylink.com/`

This site has extensive information and links to many aspects of product safety.

Public Health and Safety

`http://www.yahoo.com/Health/Public_Health_And_Safety/`

At this site, find references to public health and safety issues include, disasters, EMF health issues, fire protection, fluoridation, helmets, institutions, law enforcement, lead poisoning, lifesaving/lifeguarding, magazines, organizations, safety products, and much more.

U.S. Environmental Protection Agency

`http://www.epa.gov/`

This site contains a wealth of information about the agency and environmental issues as well as links to many other environmental and safety resources.

Self-Help and Self-Care

Healthfinder

http://www.healthfinder.gov/

Healthfinder is a gateway consumer health information Web site from the United States government. Healthfinder can lead you to selected online publications, databases, Web sites, and support and self-help groups, as well as the government agencies and nonprofit organizations that produce reliable health information for the public.

The Life Extension Foundation

http://www.lef.org/

The Life Extension Foundation is dedicated to the pursuit of a longer, healthier lifespan. Members are provided with information about the latest life extension research, products, and therapies.

LifeMatters

http://lifematters.com/index.html

LifeMatters is a very interesting site that describes itself as an ongoing conversation about taking charge of one's health and well-being for a life that is empowered, fulfilled, and profoundly related.

Personal Development Central

http://www.personal-development.com/

Find links to many journals, organizations, networks, businesses, and other information sources dealing with personal development.

Psychology Self-Help Resources on the Internet

http://www.gasou.edu/psychweb/resource/selfhelp.htm

This site contains links to non-commercial sites providing information and help about specific disorders related to psychology. It has excellent and extensive resources.

Web Links for Medical and Mental Health Problems

http://www.realtime.net/~mmjw/

An excellent source for many resources and links in many areas of medical and mental health, this site has been rated in the top five percent of all Web sites.

Whole Person Associates

http://www.wholeperson.com/wpa/index/selfhelp.htm

Self Help section of this website designed for stress and wellness specialists.

Stress Management

The American Institute of Stress

http://www.stress.org/

The homepage for the the Institute that is "Dedicated to Advancing Our Knowledge of the Role of Stress in Health and Disease."

The Anxiety-Panic Internet Resource

http://www.algy.com/anxiety/anxiety.html

This page gathers information of interest to those with the characteristic symptoms of debilitating anxiety, panic attacks, phobias, obsessive thoughts, and/or depression.

How to Fight and Conquer Stress

http://www.coolware.com/health/joel/stress.html

This is an information page on stress as it affects us and some ideas on how to deal with it.

Introduction to Stress Management, NLP, and Hypnotherapy

http://www.trance.dircon.co.uk/

This page includes a link to more good information on managing stress before it manages you.

Relax.Calm

http://weber.edu/hp/Faculty/molpin/relax/relax.html

This Stress Management Website is designed to give you resources that can help you manage your stress more effectively. It contains excellent links, great resources, and some valuable tips and guidelines that will certainly appeal to you as you are trying to find a healthy balance in these stressful times.

StressFreeNET

http://www.stressfree.com/

StressFree Network is a system of Health Care professionals providing Solutions to Stress. They provide confidential assistance to individuals, business and occupational groups for whom stress is an important issue.

Stress Management Tips for Stressed and Overworked People

http://www.stresstips.com/

This site helps you learn how to "take a practical approach to stress management. Our stress management techniques will show you how to become immune to stress...in other words how to become STRESS MANAGEMENT TOUGH."

The Web's Stress Management and Emotional Wellness Page

http://imt.net/~randolfi/StressPage.html

This is a great resource for stress management, including some excellent links and ideas for managing stress.

Tobacco, Alcohol, and Drug Use

AIRSPACE Non-smokers' Rights Society

http://airspace.bc.ca/

AIRSPACE's goals are to require all indoor public places be smoke-free, to prohibit the sale of tobacco to minors, to prohibit all forms of tobacco promotion, and to hold the tobacco industry accountable for the disease and death caused by their product.

Al-Anon and Alateen

http://www.Al-Anon-Alateen.org/

AL-ANON (and ALATEEN for younger members) is a worldwide organization that offers a self-help recovery program for families and friends of alcoholics, whether or not the alcoholic seeks help or even recognizes the existence of a drinking problem.

Center for Alcohol and Addiction Studies

http://center.butler.brown.edu/

Located at Brown University, the Center's mission is to promote the identification, prevention and effective treatment of alcohol and other drug use problems in our society through research, publications, education, and training.

Drinking: A student's guide

http://www.glness.com/ndhs/

Student's information resource on alcohol.

Drug-Related Network Resources

http://hyperreal.com/drugs/faqs/resources.html

This large list of links to many sites related to drugs of all types includes information on both sides of the controversies surrounding drugs.

Erowid's Psychoactive Vaults

http://www.erowid.org/psychoactives/psychoactives.shtml

This is a huge resource list of links to many sites related to drugs of all types. Includes information on both sides of the controversies surrounding drugs.

Facts on Tap

http://www.factsontap.org/

All the information you will ever need on alcohol and the college experience.

Join Together Online

http://www.jointogether.org/jto/

Join Together Online is the home page of a national resource center and meeting place for communities working to reduce substance abuse (illicit drugs, excessive alcohol, tobacco) and gun violence.

National Clearinghouse for Alcohol and Drug Information

http://www.health.org/

This is the information service of the Center for Substance Abuse Prevention of the U.S. Department of Health and Human Services. NCADI is the world's largest resource for current information and materials concerning substance abuse prevention.

National Institute on Drug Abuse

http://www.nida.nih.gov/

This Web site with information on the NIDA includes its organizations, calendar of events, communications, grants, and links to other related Web sites.

National Inhalant Prevention Coalition

http://www.inhalants.com/

This comprehensive page is devoted to disseminating accurate information about inhalants.

The Nicotine and Tobacco Network

http://www.nicnet.org/

This great resource from the University of Arizona contains links and information on research, news, programs, resources, and other items relating to nicotine and tobacco.

Smoking from All Sides

http://www.cs.brown.edu/people/lsh/smoking.html

Find links to Web sites on many aspects of smoking including, health aspects, statistics, tobacco news, anti-smoking groups, smoking cessation, tobacco history, commentary, pro-smoking documents, smoking glamour, and others.

Tobacco BBS

http://www.tobacco.org/

This resource center focusing on tobacco and smoking issues features tobacco news and information, assistance for smokers trying to quit, as well as a wide spectrum of tobacco-related concerns. It also offers a unique list of links to tobacco-related art, books, films, and anti-smoking activism.

Tobacco Facts Website

http://www.tobaccofacts.org/

An excellent site related to many facts and resources regarding tobacco use.

Tobacco Research Center

http://www.hsc.wvu.edu/mbrcc/trc/trc_home.htm

The TRC is an invaluable resource both for programs of national and even international impact and for individuals engaged in a personal effort to overcome nicotine addiction.

Violence

Against Domestic Violence Webring

http://www.phenomenalwomen.com/help/webring/

This site contains over 140 individual websites on violence

Canadian Women's Internet Association: Violence Against Women Information

http://www.herplace.org/violence/

Contained in this site are some very powerful articles about violence against women.

CAVNET: Communities Against Violence Network

`http://www.cavnet2.org/`

This site provides both violence information and support.

Domestic Violence Articles

`http://www.s-t.com/projects/DomVio/domviohome.HTML`

This site contains a series on violence published in 1995 by the Standard-Times of Massachusetts

Family Violence Prevention Fund

`http://www.fvpf.org/`

This is a national non-profit organization with research and outreach services.

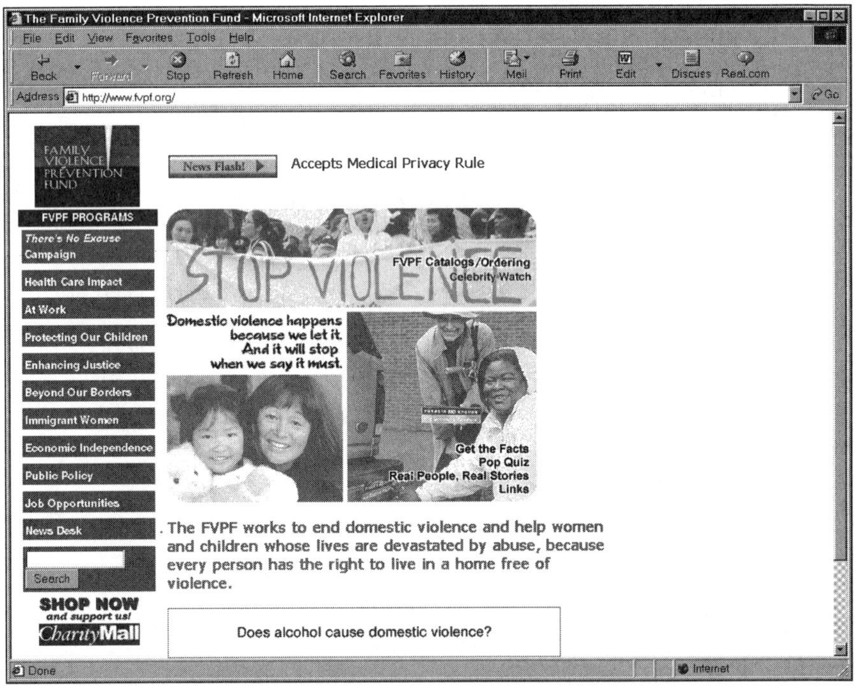

Higher Education Center Against Violence and Abuse (U. of Minn.)

`http://www.umn.edu/mincava/`

An electronic clearinghouse on violence and abuse.

Kathy's Essential Information on Abuse, Assault, Rape, & Domestic Violence

`http://www.mcs.net/~kathyw/abuse.html`

Essential Information on Abuse, Assault, Rape & Domestic Violence

Men's Issues WWW Library

`http://www.vix.com/pub/men/domestic-index.html`

Men & Domestic Violence Index.

National Crisis Prevention Institute's Violence Prevention Resource Center

`http://www.crisisprevention.com/`

CPI offers training in the safe management of disruptive and assaultive behavior.

OSHA Guidelines for Workplace Violence Prevention Programs

`http://www.osha-slc.gov/OshDoc/Additional.html`

This site contains several articles relating to worksite violence.

SafetyNet: Domestic Violence Resources

`http://www.cybergrrl.com/fs.jhtml?/views/dv/`

An International Network of Anti-Violence Experts and Advocates

U.S. Department of Justice (DOJ): Violence Against Women Office

`http://www.ojp.usdoj.gov/vawo/`

Developing the nation's capacity to prevent and control crime

Violence Against Women: Research on the Web

http://trochim.human.cornell.edu/gallery/ward/testpage.htm

A violence resource directory from Kristen Ward of Cornell University.

Weight Control

Ask the Dietitian/Overweight

http://www.dietitian.com/overweig.html

This is an excellent question-and-answer page relating to weight control, nutrition, and activity.

Food and Nutrition Information Center

http://www.nal.usda.gov/fnic/cgi-bin/ffp.pl/fnic/etext/000060.html

Outstanding resource site for all things related to weight control and obesity

Healthy Weight

http://64.58.70.236/

This Web site provides consumers, health care professionals and the media with valuable resources for weight management and healthy living. It contains related news, links, and a newsletter. It is an excellent resource.

HeliosHealth.com

http://helioshealth.com/weight_control/adult_obesity/index.html

Excellent information and resource site on obesity and weight control.

Mike Myers Medical Information on Obesity Website

http://www.weight.com/

This site provides objective medical information on obesity, eating disorders, and associated medical conditions in a non-commercial environment

Shape Up America

http://www.shapeup.org/

This web site is designed to provide you with the latest information about safe weight management and physical fitness.

What is Obesity?

http://www.weight.com/comprehensive.html

This page contains a discussion on how to lose weight permanently.

Wellness and Optimum Health

The Mind/Body Medical Institute at Harvard Medical School

http://mindbody.harvard.edu/

Find extensive information at this resource page of the Harvard Mind/ Body Clinic.

National Wellness Institute

http://www.wellnessnwi.org/

This is the home page for the National Wellness Institute, including the departments and conferences associated with it.

Wellness Web

http://www.wellweb.com/

Don Ardell's outstanding resource page on all things to do with high level wellness.

Wellness Junction

http://www.wellnessjunction.com/

Where the health information and wellness needs of consumers and professionals meet

Wellspring Wellness Newsletter

http://www.wellmedia.com/news.html

This newsletter contains interesting weekly news articles that relate to our well-being.

Women's Health

Atlanta Reproductive Health Centre

http://www.ivf.com/

This site has excellent resources for topics of interest to women. It is one of the best out there.

Breastfeeding Articles and Resources

http://www.parentsplace.com/expert/lactation/basics/

This page includes articles and information on nearly every question anyone could ever ask regarding breastfeeding.

Estronaut

http://www.womenshealth.org/

A forum for Women's health.

Melpomene Institute for Women's Health Research

http://www.melpomene.org/

This nonprofit Minneapolis-based institute, named for the first female marathon runner, specializes in health issues affecting physically active women. This Web site features topics geared to active girls and women of all ages, such as exercise during pregnancy, body image, osteoporosis, and menopause.

National Women's Health Information Center

http://www.4woman.gov/

The National Women's Health Information Center is a one-stop gateway for women seeking health information. NWHIC is a free information and resource service on women's health issues designed just for you, whether you're a consumer, a health care professional, a researcher, an educator, or a student.

Sexual Assault Information

http://www.cs.utk.edu/~bartley/saInfoPage.html

This page includes a nice search for many subtopics falling under the main topic of sexual assault. This is an excellent reference.

Women's Health Information

http://www.yahoo.com/Health/Women_s_Health/

This is a Yahoo! search for all things on the Internet related to women's health.

Women's Health Interactive

http://www.womens-health.com/

A site whose mission is to empower women through knowledge and action.

part 3

Documentation

Your Citation for Exemplary Research

There's another detail left for us to handle—the formal citing of electronic sources in academic papers. The very factor that makes research on the Internet exciting is the same factor that makes referencing these sources challenging: their dynamic nature. A journal article exists, either in print or on microfilm, virtually forever. A document on the Internet can come, go, and change without warning. Because the purpose of citing sources is to allow another scholar to retrace your argument, a good citation allows a reader to obtain information from your primary sources, to the extent possible. This means you need to include not only information on when a source was posted on the Internet (if available) but also when you obtained the information.

The two arbiters of form for academic and scholarly writing are the Modern Language Association (MLA) and the American Psychological Association (APA); both organizations have established styles for citing electronic publications.

MLA Style

In the fifth edition of the *MLA Handbook for Writers of Research Papers,* the MLA recommends the following formats:

- **URLs:** URLs are enclosed in angle brackets (<>) and contain the access mode identifier, the formal name for such indicators as "http" or "ftp." If a URL must be split across two lines, break it only after a slash (/). Never introduce a hyphen at the end of the first line. The URL should include all the parts necessary to identify uniquely the file/document being cited.

  <http://www.csun.edu/~rtvfdept/home/index.html>

- **An online scholarly project or reference database:** A complete online reference contains the title of the project or database (underlined); the name of the editor of the project or database (if given); electronic publication information, including version number (if relevant and if not part of the title), date of electronic publication or latest update, and name of any sponsoring institution or organization; date of access; and electronic address.

The Perseus Project. Ed. Gregory R. Crane. Mar. 1997. Department of Classics, Tufts University. 15 June 1998 <http://www.perseus.tufts.edu/>.

If you cannot find some of the information, then include the information that is available. The MLA also recommends that you print or download electronic documents, freezing them in time for future reference.

- **A document within a scholarly project or reference database:** It is much more common to use only a portion of a scholarly project or database. To cite an essay, poem, or other short work, begin this citation with the name of the author and the title of the work (in quotation marks). Then, include all the information used when citing a complete online scholarly project or reference database, however, make sure you use the URL of the specific work and not the address of the general site.

Cuthberg, Lori. "Moonwalk: Earthlings' Finest Hour." Discovery Channel Online. 1999. Discovery Channel. 25 Nov. 1999 <http://www.discovery.com/indep/newsfeatures/moonwa lk/challenge.html>.

- **A professional or personal site:** Include the name of the person creating the site (reversed), followed by a period, the title of the site (underlined), or, if there is no title, a description such as Home page (such a description is neither placed in quotes nor underlined). Then, specify the name of any school, organization, or other institution affiliated with the site and follow it with your date of access and the URL of the page.

```
Packer, Andy. Home page. 1 Apr. 1998 <http://
   www.suu.edu/~students/Packer.htm>.
```

Some electronic references are truly unique to the online domain. These include email, newsgroup postings, MUDs (multiuser domains) or MOOs (multiuser domains, object-oriented), and IRCs (Internet Relay Chats).

Email In citing email messages, begin with the writer's name (reversed) followed by a period, then the title of the message (if any) in quotations as it appears in the subject line. Next comes a description of the message, typically "Email to," and the recipient (e.g., "the author"), and finally the date of the message.


```
Davis, Jeffrey. "Web Writing Resources." Email to
   Nora Davis. 3 Jan. 2000.

Sommers, Laurice. "Re: College Admissions Practices."
   Email to the author. 12 Aug. 1998.
```

List Servers and Newsgroups In citing these references, begin with the author's name (reversed) followed by a period. Next include the title of the document (in quotes) from the subject line, followed by the words "Online posting" (not in quotes). Follow this with the date of posting. For list servers, include the date of access, the name of the list (if known), and the online address of the list's moderator or administrator. For newsgroups, follow "Online posting" with the date of posting, the date of access, and the name of the newsgroup, prefixed with "news:" and enclosed in angle brackets.

```
Applebaum, Dale. "Educational Variables." Online
   posting. 29 Jan. 1998. Higher Education
   Discussion Group. 30 Jan. 1993
   <jlucidoj@unc.edu>.

Gostl, Jack. "Re: Mr. Levitan." Online posting.
   13 June 1997. 20 June 1997
   <news:alt.edu.bronxscience>.
```

MUDs, MOOs, and IRCs Begin with the name of the speaker(s) followed by a period. Follow with the description and date of the event, the forum in which the communication took place, the date of access, and the online address. If you accessed the MOO or MUD through telnet, your citation might appear as follows:

```
Guest. Personal interview. 13 Aug. 1998. <telnet://
   du.edu:8888>.
```

For more information on MLA documentation style for online sources, check out their Web site at http://www.mla.org/style/sources.htm.

APA Style

part 3

The *Publication Manual of the American Psychological Association* (4th ed.) is fairly dated in its handling of online sources, having been published before the rise of the WWW and the generally recognized format for URLs. The format that follows is based on the APA manual, with modifications. It's important to remember that, unlike the MLA, the APA does not include temporary or transient sources (e.g., letters, phone calls, etc.) in its "References" page, preferring to handle them in in-text citations exclusively. This rule holds for electronic sources as well: email, MOOs/MUDs, list server postings, etc., are not included in the "References" page, merely cited in text, for example, "But Wilson has rescinded his earlier support for these policies" (Charles Wilson, personal email to the author, 20 November 1996). But also note that many list server and Usenet groups and MOOs actually archive their correspondences, so that there is a permanent site (usually a Gopher or FTP server) where those documents reside. In that case, you would want to find the archive and cite it as an unchanging source. Strictly speaking, according to the APA manual, a file from an FTP site should be referenced as follows:

```
Deutsch, P. (1991). Archie: An electronic directory
   service for the Internet [Online]. Available
   FTP: ftp.sura.net Directory: pub/archie/docs File:
   whatis.archie.
```

However, the increasing familiarity of Net users with the convention of a URL makes the prose description of how to find a file ("Available FTP: ftp.sura.net Directory: pub/archie/docs File: whatis.archie") unnecessary.

So, with modification of the APA format (as suggested by the APA at its Web page www.apa.org/journals/webref.html), citations from the standard Internet sources would appear as follows.

FTP (File Transfer Protocol) Sites To cite files available for downloading via FTP, give the author's name (if known), the publication date (if available and if different from the date accessed), the full title of the paper (capitalizing only the first word and proper nouns), the date of access, and the address of the FTP site along with the full path necessary to access the file.

Deutsch, P. (1991) Archie: An electronic directory service for the Internet. Retrieved January 25, 2000 from File Transfer Protocol: ftp://ftp.sura.net/pub/archie/docs/whatis.archie

WWW Sites (World Wide Web) To cite files available for viewing or downloading via the World Wide Web, give the author's name (if known), the year of publication (if known and if different from the date accessed), the full title of the article, and the title of the complete work (if applicable) in italics. Include any additional information (such as versions, editions, or revisions) in parentheses immediately following the title. Include the date of retrieval and full URL (the http address).

Burka, L. P. (1993). A hypertext history of multi-user dungeons. *MUDdex*. Retrieved January 13, 1997 from the World Wide Web: http://www.utopia.com/talent/lpb/muddex/essay/

Tilton, J. (1995). Composing good HTML (Vers. 2.0.6). Retrieved December 1, 1996 from the World Wide Web: http://www.cs.cmu.edu/~tilt/cgh/

Synchronous Communications (MOOs, MUDs, IRC, etc.) Give the name of the speaker(s), the complete date of the conversation being referenced in parentheses, and the title of the session (if applicable). Next, list the title of the site in italics, the protocol and address (if applicable), and any directions necessary to access the work. Last, list the date of access, followed by the retrieval information. Personal interviews do not need to be listed in the References, but do need to be included in parenthetic references in the text (see the APA *Publication Manual*).

Cross, J. (1996, February 27). Netoric's Tuesday cafe: Why use MUDs in the writing classroom? *MediaMoo.* Retrieved March 1, 1996 from File Transfer Protocol: ftp://daedalus.com/pub/ACW/NETORIC/catalog

Gopher Sites List the author's name (if applicable), the year of publication, the title of the file or paper, and the title of the complete work (if applicable). Include any print publication information (if available) followed by the protocol (i.e., gopher://). List the date that the file was accessed and the path necessary to access the file.

Massachusetts Higher Education Coordinating Council. (1994). Using coordination and collaboration to address change. Retrieved July 16, 1999 from the World Wide Web: gopher://gopher.mass.edu:170/00gopher_root%3A%5B_hecc%5D_plan

Email, Listservs, and Newsgroups Do not include personal email in the list of References. Although unretrievable communication such as email is not included in APA References, somewhat more public or accessible Internet postings from newsgroups or listservs may be included. See the APA *Publication Manual* for information on in-text citations.

Heilke, J. (1996, May 3). Webfolios. Alliance for Computers and Writing Discussion List. Retrieved December 31, 1996 from the World Wide Web: http://www.ttu.edu/lists/acw-l/9605/0040.html

Other authors and educators have proposed similar extensions to the APA style. You can find links to these pages at:

www.psychwww.com/resource/apacrib.htm

Remember, "frequently-referenced" does not equate to "correct" or even "desirable." Check with your professor to see if your course or school has a preference for an extended APA style.

appendix

List of URLs (Web Addresses)

Health News

http://abcnews.go.com/sections/Living/
http://www.achoo.com/news/default.asp
http://aol.drkoop.com/news/
http://www.all-natural.com/news.html
http://www.eatright.org/news/
http://www.chronicillnet.org/online/
http://cnn.com/HEALTH/index.html
http://health.discovery.com/
http://healthanswers.com/News/News.asp
http://www.healthcentral.com/news/news.cfm
http://www.ljextra.com/practice/health/index.html
http://www.trufax.org/menu/health1.html
http://www.intelihealth.com/IH/ihtIH/WSIHW000/333/333.html
http://www.lentilhealth.com/
http://www.mayohealth.org/home
http://www.msnbc.com/news/HEALTH_Front.asp?a
http://www.nandotimes.com/noframes/healthscience/
http://www.health.org/newsroom/
http://www.newsrx.net/dailynews.cgi
http://www.npr.org/news/healthsci/
http://www.reutershealth.com/
http://www.sciencedaily.com/index.htm
http://www.medicinenet.com/Script/Main/HP.asp?li=USA&d=110&cu=16583&w=0
http://webmd.lycos.com/headlines/
http://www.wellmedia.com/news.html

http://www.yahoo.com/headlines/health/
http://199.97.97.16/contWriter/yhd7/

Health Related Searches

http://www.100hot.com/directory/sports/health.html
http://home.about.com/health/index.htm?IN2PID=938983637.500418&IN2ID=938983637.500418
http://altavista.looksmart.com/eus1/eus53940/r?l&izf&
http://www.aj.com/main/askjeeves.asp?ask=health&origin=&site_name=Jeeves&metasearch=yes
http://www.dmoz.org/Health/
http://catalog.dogpile.com/texis/catalog?c=Health
http://www.webdirectory.com/Health/
http://my.excite.com/lifestyle/health_and_fitness/
http://www.einet.net/galaxy/Community/Health.html
http://www.go2net.com/channels/health/
http://www.go.com/Center/Health?svx=CTOC_Health
http://www.google.com/search?q=health
http://www.healthatoz.com/
http://guide-p.infoseek.com/Health?tid=1207
http://www.looksmart.com/eus1/eus317837/eus317920/r?comefrom=nspanel-eus317920
http://dir.lycos.com/Health/
http://magellan.excite.com/health
http://metahoo.com/cgi-bin/apexec.pl?etype=odp&template=smart.htm&passurl=/Health/
http://www.medexplorer.com/
http://directory.netscape.com/Health/?cp=srpmatcat
http://www.northernlight.com/nlquery.fcg?cb=0&qr=health&orl=
http://www.snap.com/directory/category/0%2C16%2C-7%2C00.html?st.sn.fd.0.dir-7
http://www.stpt.com/channel.asp?id=4
http://vh.radiology.uiowa.edu/Misc/Search.html
http://webcrawler.com/Health/
http://www.yahoo.com/Health/

Health Related Journals, Magazines, and Periodicals

http://www.forthrt.com/~chronicl/homepage.html
http://www.fitnessworld.com
http://www.lifelines.com/newsletter/frame.html
http://www.medscape.com/

http://www.medscape.com/Home/Topics/multispecialty/directories/dir-MULT.JournalRoom.html
http://www.mensfitness.com/
http://www.newage.com/
http://www.newfrontier.com/
http://www.nejm.org/
http://www.cspinet.org/nah/
http://www.physsportsmed.com/
http://www.shareguide.com/mag/
http://www.yogajournal.com/

Health Research and Evaluation

http://www.carl.org/Access.html
http://chid.nih.gov/
http://it.usu.edu/itrs/AEA/index.html
http://ericae.net/
http://www.findarticles.com/PI/index.jhtml
http://www.healthfinder.gov/moretools/
http://www.healthgate.com/
http://www.healthgate.com/HealthGate/MEDLINE/search.shtml
http://www.nyu.edu/education/hepr/resources/online/index.html
http://web.indstate.edu/hlthsfty/ch/bkmrks.htm

Alternative Medicine and Holistic Health

http://www.Acupuncture.com/
http://www.amfoundation.org/
http://www.pitt.edu/~cbw/altm.html
http://www.altmedicine.com/
http://www.americanwholehealth.com/
http://ahha.org/
http://www.amtamassage.org/
http://www.dreamup.com/
http://www.kcweb.com/herb/herbmain.htm
http://www.herbnet.com/
http://www.herbs.org/index.html
http://www.holisticmed.com/
http://www.homeopathyhome.com/
http://www.iahf.com/
http://www.nderf.org/
http://nccam.nih.gov/
http://www.oxytherapy.com/

http://www.spiritweb.org/
http://wellmedia.com/links.html

Cancer

http://www.cancer.org/
http://www.aicr.org/
http://www.cancercareinc.org/
http://www.cancernews.com/
http://www.uri.edu/research/cprc/
http://www.cansearch.org/canserch/canserch.htm
http://www.ncl.ac.uk/~nchwww/guides/clinks1.htm
http://www.jomol.regensburg.com/
http://cancernet.nci.nih.gov/pdqfull.html
http://www.cancer.med.umich.edu/NCCN/NCCN.html
http://www.maui.net/~southsky/introto.html
http://cancerguide.org/
http://www.oncolink.upenn.edu/
http://www.yahoo.com/Health/Diseases_and_Conditions/Cancer/

Community Health Education

http://www.americanheart.org/
http://www.cdc.gov/cdc.html
http://web.indstate.edu/hlthsfty/ch/ch.htm
http://ctb.lsi.ukans.edu/
http://userwww.service.emory.edu/~cescoff/cam.html
http://www.cdc.gov/nchs/about.htm
http://nhic-nt.health.org/
http://www.nih.gov/
http://www.homepage.holowww.com/
http://www.paho.org/
http://www.who.ch/

Diseases: Chronic and Acute

http://www.diabetes.org/
http://www.lungusa.org/
http://www.cdc.gov/
http://www.chronicillnet.org/

http://www.ohsu.edu/cliniweb/C.html
http://www.mic.ki.se/Diseases/index.html
http://medhlp.netusa.net/
http://www.cdc.gov/epo/mmwr/mmwr.html
http://www.mothernature.com/
http://www3.bc.sympatico.ca/me/patientsguide/
http://www.virusmyth.com/aids/index.htm
http://www.bocklabs.wisc.edu/Welcome.html
http://my.webmd.com/condition_center_all
http://www.yahoo.com/Health/Diseases_and_Conditions/

Environmental Health

http://atsdr1.atsdr.cdc.gov:8080/cx.html
http://www.cdc.gov/nceh/ncehhome.htm
http://www.niehs.nih.gov/
http://www.pacificrim.net/~nature/
http://www.yahoo.com/Health/Environmental_Health/

Exercise and Fitness

http://www.aahperd.org/
http://www.acsm.org/
http://www.acefitness.org/
http://www.cascade.org/links.html
http://www.clark.net/pub/pribut/spsport.html
http://www.noah.cuny.edu/pregnancy/march_of_dimes/pre_preg.plan/fit42is.html
http://www.sportlink.com/fitness/
http://www.ncppa.org/
http://home.ait.ac.nz/staff/pmellow//
http://www.physsportsmed.com/
http://www.rrca.org/
http://sunsite.unc.edu/drears/running/running.html
http://www.runnersworld.com/
http://fiat.gslis.utexas.edu/~lewisa/womsprt.html

General Health

http://www.aol.com/webcenters/health/home.adp
http://www.clearinghouse.net/cgi-bin/chadmin/viewcat/Health___Medicine?kywd++

http://h-devil-www.mc.duke.edu/h-devil
http://www.cc.columbia.edu/cu/healthwise/
http://www.arcade.uiowa.edu/hardin-www/md.html
http://healthanswers.com/
http://www.healthtouch.com/
http://www.healthy.net/
http://www.intelihealth.com/IH/
ihtIH?t=408&st=408&r=WSIHW000
http://www.kidshealth.org/index2.html
http://www.northwesternmutual.com/games/longevity/
http://www.mediconsult.com/
http://www.ncahf.org/
http://www3.bc.sympatico.ca/me/patientsguide/
http://www.youfirst.com/

Governmental Health Resources

http://www.acf.dhhs.gov/
http://www.hhs.gov/
http://www.fda.gov/
http://www.hcfa.gov/
http://www.hrsa.dhhs.gov/
http://www.health.gov/healthypeople/
http://www.nlm.nih.gov/

Health and Disease Care

http://www.amso.com/
http://www.centerwatch.com/
http://www.convergentmedical.com/
http://www.globalmedic.com/
http://www.life-line.org/
http://www.medscape.com/Home/About.html
http://www.yahoo.com/Health/Health_Care/

Health Education (School)

http://www.ericsp.org/
http://www.ericsp.org/pages/healthpe/index.html
http://eta.aed.org/

http://www.ex.ac.uk/~dregis/healthy.html
http://www.pecentral.org/lessonideas/health/healthlp.html

Health Organizations

http://www.aahperd.org/
http://www.aarp.org/
http://www.acha.org/
http://www.ashaweb.org/
http://www.awhp.org/

Health Promotion

http://www.awhp.org/
http://www.ihpr.ubc.ca/
http://www.monash.edu.au/health/
http://odphp.osophs.dhhs.gov/
http://www.siu.edu/~crhssd/rhres.htm
http://www.welcoa.org/

Health Psychology

http://www.recovery.org/aa/
http://www.apa.org/
http://www.concentric.net/~conure/allen.html
http://www.athealth.com/
http://www.shef.ac.uk/~psysc/psychotherapy/index.html
http://www.uwsp.edu/acad/psych/dk/danielpg.htm
http://www.infinityinst.com/
http://fly.hiwaay.net/~garson/
http://www.mentalhealth.com/main.html
http://www.cmhc.com/
http://mentalhealth.about.com/health/mentalhealth/library/blsearch.htm
http://www.cloud9.net/~thorpy/
http://www.nerdworld.com/users/dstein/nw142.html
http://www.clas.ufl.edu/users/gthursby/taoism/
http://www.rider.edu/users/suler/zenstory/zenstory.html

Heart Health

http://www.americanheart.org/
http://www.cardio.com/articles/preventn.htm
http://www.cardio.com/
http://www.fi.edu/biosci/heart.html
http://sln.fi.edu/biosci/healthy/healthy.html
http://www.mindspring.com/~mtm/news.html
http://www.hsforum.com/frameset1.asp?loc=learningctr.asp
http://www.internetwks.com/pauling/
http://www.fatfree.com/FAQ/ada-paper

Nutrition

http://www.eatright.org/
http://www.americanheart.org/catalog/Health_catpage4.html
http://arborcom.com/
http://www.dietitian.com/
http://www.holisticmed.com/aspartame/
http://www1.mhv.net/~donn/diet.html
http://www.cspinet.org/
http://www.cyberdiet.com/
http://www.globalgourmet.com/
http://www.olen.com/food/
http://www.nalusda.gov/fnic/
http://www.ganesa.com/food/index.html
http://dinnercoop.cs.cmu.edu/dinnercoop/special/health.html
http://ificinfo.health.org/
http://www.mymenus.com/
http://www.nutrition.gov/home/index.php3
http://www.nutribase.com/
http://academic.brooklyn.cuny.edu/hns/prins/
http://www.vegweb.com/

Public Health

http://www.apha.org/
http://www.sph.emory.edu/studentservice/Career.html
http://www.newsrx.net/home.cgi
http://www-sci.lib.uci.edu/~martindale/PHealth.html

Safety and Injury Prevention

http://www.webdirectory.com/
http://www.bhsi.org/index.htm
gopher://cpsc.gov/
http://www.injurypreventionweb.org/
http://www.niehs.nih.gov/
http://www.cdc.gov/niosh/homepage.html
http://www.nsc.org/
http://www.safetylink.com/
http://www.yahoo.com/Health/Public_Health_And_Safety/
http://www.epa.gov/

Self-Help and Self-Care

http://www.healthfinder.gov/
http://www.lef.org/
http://lifematters.com/index.html
http://www.personal-development.com/
http://www.gasou.edu/psychweb/resource/selfhelp.htm
http://www.realtime.net/~mmjw/
http://www.wholeperson.com/wpa/index/selfhelp.htm

Stress Management

http://www.stress.org/
http://www.algy.com/anxiety/anxiety.html
http://www.coolware.com/health/joel/stress.html
http://www.trance.dircon.co.uk/
http://weber.edu/hp/Faculty/molpin/relax/relax.html
http://www.stressfree.com/
http://www.stresstips.com/
http://imt.net/~randolfi/StressPage.html

Tobacco, Alcohol, and Drug Use

http://airspace.bc.ca/
http://www.Al-Anon-Alateen.org/

http://center.butler.brown.edu/
http://www.glness.com/ndhs/
http://hyperreal.com/drugs/faqs/resources.html
http://www.erowid.org/psychoactives/psychoactives.shtml
http://www.factsontap.org/
http://www.jointogether.org/jto/
http://www.health.org/
http://www.nida.nih.gov/
http://www.inhalants.com/
http://www.nicnet.org/
http://www.cs.brown.edu/people/lsh/smoking.html
http://www.tobacco.org/
http://www.tobaccofacts.org/
http://www.hsc.wvu.edu/mbrcc/trc/trc_home.htm

Violence

http://www.phenomenalwomen.com/help/webring/
http://www.herplace.org/violence/
http://www.cavnet2.org/
http://www.s-t.com/projects/DomVio/domviohome.HTML
http://www.fvpf.org/
http://www.umn.edu/mincava/
http://www.mcs.net/~kathyw/abuse.html
http://www.vix.com/pub/men/domestic-index.html
http://www.crisisprevention.com/
http://www.osha-slc.gov/OshDoc/Additional.html
http://www.cybergrrl.com/fs.jhtml?/views/dv/
http://www.ojp.usdoj.gov/vawo/
http://trochim.human.cornell.edu/gallery/ward/testpage.htm

Weight Control

http://www.dietitian.com/overweig.html
http://www.nal.usda.gov/fnic/cgi-bin/ffp.pl/fnic/etext/000060.html
http://64.58.70.236/
http://helioshealth.com/weight_control/adult_obesity/index.html
http://www.weight.com/
http://www.shapeup.org/
http://www.weight.com/comprehensive.html

Wellness and Optimum Health

http://mindbody.harvard.edu/
http://www.wellnessnwi.org/
http://www.wellweb.com/
http://www.wellnessjunction.com/
http://www.wellmedia.com/news.html

Women's Health

http://www.ivf.com/
http://www.parentsplace.com/expert/lactation/basics/
http://www.womenshealth.org/
http://www.melpomene.org/
http://www.4woman.gov/
http://www.cs.utk.edu/~bartley/saInfoPage.html
http://www.yahoo.com/Health/Women_s_Health/
http://www.womens-health.com/

Glossary

Your Own Private Glossary

The Glossary in this book contains reference terms you'll find useful as you get started on the Internet. After a while, however, you'll find yourself running across abbreviations, acronyms, and buzzwords whose definitions will make more sense to you once you're no longer a novice (or "newbie"). That's the time to build a glossary of your own. For now, the 2DNet Webopædia gives you a place to start.

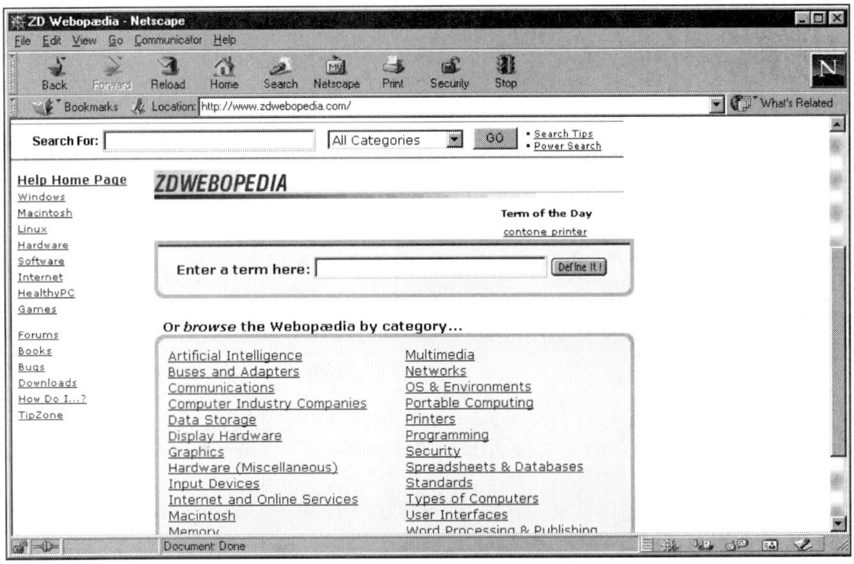

alias
A simple email address that can be used in place of a more complex one.

AVI
Audio Video Interleave. A video compression standard developed for use with Microsoft Windows. Video clips on the World Wide Web are usually available in both AVI and QuickTime formats.

bandwidth
Internet parlance for capacity to carry or transfer information such as email and Web pages.

browser
The computer program that lets you view the contents of Web sites.

client
A program that runs on your personal computer and supplies you with Internet services, such as getting your mail.

cyberspace
The whole universe of information that is available from computer networks. The term was coined by science fiction writer William Gibson in his novel *Neuromancer,* published in 1984.

DNS
See *domain name server.*

domain
A group of computers administered as a single unit, typically belonging to a single organization such as a university or corporation.

domain name
A name that identifies one or more computers belonging to a single domain. For example, “apple.com”.

domain name server
A computer that converts domain names into the numeric addresses used on the Internet.

download
Copying a file from another computer to your computer over the Internet.

email
Electronic mail.

emoticon
A guide to the writer’s feelings, represented by typed characters, such as the Smiley :-). Helps readers understand the emotions underlying a written message.

FAQs
Frequently Asked Questions

flame
A rude or derogatory message directed as a personal attack against an individual or group.

flame war
An exchange of flames (see above).

FTP
File Transfer Protocol, a method of moving files from one computer to another over the Internet.

home page
A page on the World Wide Web that acts as a starting point for information about a person or organization.

hypertext
Text that contains embedded *links* to other pages of text. Hypertext enables the reader to navigate between pages of related information by following links in the text.

LAN
Local Area Network. A computer network that is located in a concentrated area, such as offices within a building.

link
A reference to a location on the Web that is embedded in the text of the Web page. Links are usually highlighted with a different color or underlined to make them easily visible.

listserv
Strictly speaking, a computer program that administers electronic mailing lists, but also used to denote such lists or discussion groups, as in "the writer's listserv."

lurker
A passive reader of an Internet *newsgroup* or *listserv.* A lurker reads messages, but does not participate in the discussion by posting or responding to messages.

mailing list
A subject-specific automated email system. Users subscribe and receive email from other users about the subject of the list.

modem
A device for connecting two computers over a telephone line.

newbie
A new user of the Internet.

newsgroup
A discussion forum in which all participants can read all messages and public replies between the participants.

plug-in
A third-party software program that will lend a Web browser (Netscape, Internet Explorer, etc.) additional features.

quoted
Text in an email message or newsgroup posting that has been set off by the use of vertical bars or > characters in the left-hand margin.

search engine
A computer program that will locate Web sites or files based on specified criteria.

secure
A Web page whose contents are encrypted when sending or receiving information.

server
A computer program that moves information on request, such as a Web server that sends pages to your browser.

Smiley
See *emoticon.*

snail mail
Mail sent the old fashioned way: Write a letter, put it in an envelope, stick on a stamp, and drop it in the mailbox.

spam
Spam is to the Internet as unsolicited junk mail is to the postal system.

URL
Uniform Resource Locator: The notation for specifying addresses on the World Wide Web (e.g. http://www.abacon.com or ftp://ftp.abacon.com).

Usenet
The section of the Internet devoted to *newsgroups.*

Web browser
A program used to navigate and access information on the World Wide Web. Web browsers convert html coding into a display of pictures, sound, and words.

Web page
All the text, graphics, pictures, and so forth, denoted by a single URL beginning with the identifier "http://".

Web site
A collection of World Wide Web pages, usually consisting of a home page and several other linked pages.